Simplified Phacoemulsification

Simplified Phacoemulsification

Second Edition

Navneet Toshniwal
MBBS MS (Ophthalmology)
Medical Director
Navneet Hospital
Solapur, Maharashtra, India

Forewords
SH Lee
Janet Hina

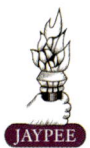

JAYPEE BROTHERS MEDICAL PUBLISHERS
The Health Sciences Publisher
New Delhi | London

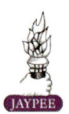 **Jaypee Brothers Medical Publishers (P) Ltd**

Headquarters
Jaypee Brothers Medical Publishers (P) Ltd
EMCA House, 23/23-B
Ansari Road, Daryaganj
New Delhi 110 002, India
Landline: +91-11-23272143, +91-11-23272703
+91-11-23282021, +91-11-23245672
Email: jaypee@jaypeebrothers.com

Corporate Office
Jaypee Brothers Medical Publishers (P) Ltd
4838/24, Ansari Road, Daryaganj
New Delhi 110 002, India
Phone: +91-11-43574357
Fax: +91-11-43574314
Email: jaypee@jaypeebrothers.com

Overseas Office
JP Medical Ltd.
83, Victoria Street, London
SW1H 0HW (UK)
Phone: +44 20 3170 8910
Fax: +44 (0)20 3008 6180
Email: info@jpmedpub.com

Website: www.jaypeebrothers.com
Website: www.jaypeedigital.com

© 2025, Jaypee Brothers Medical Publishers

The views and opinions expressed in this book are solely those of the original contributor(s)/author(s) and do not necessarily represent those of editor(s) or publisher of the book.

All rights reserved. No part of this publication may be reproduced, stored or transmitted in any form or by any means, electronic, mechanical, photocopying, recording or otherwise, without the prior permission in writing of the publishers.

All brand names and product names used in this book are trade names, service marks, trademarks or registered trademarks of their respective owners. The publisher is not associated with any product or vendor mentioned in this book.

Medical knowledge and practice change constantly. This book is designed to provide accurate, authoritative information about the subject matter in question. However, readers are advised to check the most current information available on procedures included and check information from the manufacturer of each product to be administered, to verify the recommended dose, formula, method and duration of administration, adverse effects and contraindications. It is the responsibility of the practitioner to take all appropriate safety precautions. Neither the publisher nor the author(s)/editor(s) assume any liability for any injury and/or damage to persons or property arising from or related to use of material in this book.

This book is sold on the understanding that the publisher is not engaged in providing professional medical services. If such advice or services are required, the services of a competent medical professional should be sought.

Every effort has been made where necessary to contact holders of copyright to obtain permission to reproduce copyright material. If any have been inadvertently overlooked, the publisher will be pleased to make the necessary arrangements at the first opportunity.

Inquiries for bulk sales may be solicited at: jaypee@jaypeebrothers.com

Simplified Phacoemulsification

First Edition: 2013
Second Edition: **2025**
ISBN: 978-93-5696-738-0

Printed in India at Sterling Graphics Pvt. Ltd.

Dedicated to
My dear parents
Father, late Dr Sham Toshniwal
Mother, Sou Chand Toshniwal

Foreword

Ophthalmic surgery technology has undergone rapid advancements and innovations in the last two decades. From modest and conventional surgical techniques in the early eighties, it has now become a high-tech surgery with least indoor stay and excellent visual outcomes.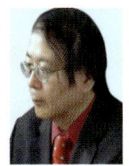

Modern phaco surgery is a vast subject. It is important for ophthalmologists to master various surgical steps in the phaco surgery procedures to ensure the best surgical result. There are very few qualities international surgical techniques in an ophthalmic book which can teach and guide the ophthalmologists to master various surgical techniques properly. Keeping this factor in view, Dr Navneet Toshniwal has conceptualized the essential and practical steps of phaco surgical techniques in ophthalmology which shall contain in this book. The book has covered all aspects of phaco surgery in a comprehensive and easy-to-read format for the benefit of ophthalmologists worldwide.

My hat goes off to Dr Navneet Toshniwal for his great effort in writing this simple and practical ophthalmic book with an innovative approach to phaco surgery.

For this reason, an ophthalmic book such as this is a valuable resource, allowing the phaco surgeons to consult the book each time they step into the operating room. I suspect that this book will find a home near operating theaters and surgical suites around the globe, and many of these chapters will become worn from the many re-readings that will occur just before procedures begin. All phaco surgeons seek to promote the best visual outcome with the least amount of surgical trauma. This book will help the surgeons to achieve this aim.

SH Lee
MD FRCS(C) FAAO
Chief
Department of Ophthalmology
Sunray Surgical Center
Vancouver, BC, Canada

Foreword

When I decided to expand my career to include phacoemulsification, I was fortunate to have Dr Navneet Toshniwal to help me go through the change, and that was incredibly rewarding.

One of the truly great things about this book is that it provides the principles of phacoemulsification in a simple way to help every ophthalmologist who wants to start his/her journey in shifting from extracapsular cataract surgery to phacoemulsification.

I congratulate and thank my colleague Dr Navneet Toshniwal for providing all this knowledge in a well-organized, informative, yet easily understood book.

Janet Hina
MD FRCS(Ed)
Consultant Pediatric Ophthalmologist
Department of Ophthalmology
Royal Medical Services
Jordan

Preface to the Second Edition

I am very happy to present the 2nd edition of this book to you. I have tried my best to put the concepts of phaco in a very precise but simplified way. This simplified approach of writing was largely appreciated by all. I have written three more books. *Text and Atlas: Slit Lamp Biomicroscopy for Assessment in Cataract Surgery* was released in 2014, *Do's and Don'ts in Phaco Surgery* in 2019 and book *Phaco Machine and Its Application* in 2022. There is a huge demand for my books not just in India but also in Africa, especially the Franco Belt, and therefore two of my books have been translated into French. This book is also under process of translation into French. The huge success of all these books motivated and encouraged me to write the 2nd edition of this book. This 2nd edition has my experiences added in a simpler way. Writing the 2nd edition was not easy, but the journey was made easy by great cooperation with M/s Jaypee Brothers Medical Publishers (P) Ltd, New Delhi, India.

Being a 2nd generation ophthalmologist, I always had guidance from my father, late Dr Sham Toshniwal. He always encouraged me to concentrate on the academic part too, along with practice. Taking the motivation and blessings from my father and his great friend Dr Vilas Salgarkar, I keep working in the academic field. Now joined by the 3rd generation of ophthalmologists—Dr Nikhil, Dr Ayushi, and Dr Sumit—I got valuable scientific inputs in writing the book.

The phaco training program, which I started in 2002, is still going on at our institute. Since 2013, it got more structured and meticulous under the banner of Navneet Academy of Ophthalmology, Solapur, Maharashtra, India. Everyday analysis of the steps of phaco surgery with trainee doctors is the core of our training program. It gives new ideas related to the subject. I gathered all these views, ideas, and concepts related to phaco in the form of notes. The sharing of knowledge and discussions with national and international ophthalmologists and ophthalmic industry legends has helped me a lot to share new, more simplified concepts in this 2nd edition.

I feel extremely happy to share this very useful and good scientific content in the most simple way with lots of self-explanatory figures to my colleagues and postgraduate students worldwide.

Navneet Toshniwal

Preface to the First Edition

I am very happy to present this book to you. I have tried my best to put concepts of phaco in very precise but simplified way. This book will give an idea of technical details of the steps of phaco. This important information is helpful to all ophthalmic surgeons, paramedical staff such as technical people related to phaco machine, nursing staff mainly operation theater assistants, simple though.

Mine is second generation of ophthalmologist in the family. I started my career in April 1994. Being second generation eye surgeon, I got opportunity to see my father Dr Sham Toshniwal since my childhood. Because of his dedicated practice in this field since 1969, I had very big impact on my mind to become a doctor and then in successive years as an eye surgeon. He is very good clinician. His practice is based on practical aspects and for patients well-being. Every day he spends some time to read journals. Apart from his practice, his keen interest is social work, so he started Blind School and Eye Bank in 1988 and developed to its top level. Dr Vilas Salgarkar who is one of the best friends of my father still comes as an Anesthesiologist to our hospital. In between surgical sessions, there is a tea break everyday at our hospital. During these intervals, many times we discuss academic aspects of ophthalmology and mainly surgical aspects. One day, during our discussion, my father mentioned that he has practiced in practical way, but he could not give time to academics. Both of them suggested me to start concentrating on academic part of ophthalmology. This advice has changed my career. I used to attend all regional, state, and national conferences very regularly, but without presentation. I started to attend International conferences since 2000. Slowly I began to present papers, videos at all level of conferences.

I have passed MBBS from Dr VM Medical College, Solapur, Maharashtra, India in 1988. I have completed my MS Ophthalmology at the same college under the able guidance of Dr MV Albal and Dr BN Bangade in 1992. In 1993–94, I have got a fellowship at Sankara Nethralaya, Chennai, Tamil Nadu, India, under guidance of Dr SS Badrinath. The way of practicing in this institute, the dedication of all consultants, approach or concern towards patients, day-to-day seminar on different topics and concept of video library in ophthalmology changed my vision and approach to look towards this subject.

Dr Nitin Prabhudesai who is my friend was behind me to start phaco in those days. First time I saw demonstration of phaco at Dr Jeevan Ladi's clinic at Pune, Maharashtra. I started my phaco practice in 1997. I was attending usually all our regional phaco workshops those days. I had a great impact of lectures and demonstrations of phaco surgery by Dr Amar Agrawal, Dr Mahipal Sachdev which were conducted at National Institute of Ophthalmology (NIO), Pune. Reading books of Dr Shashi Kapoor and these doctors had a great impact on me. I also had a great impact of surgical work of Dr Abhay Vasvda, Dr KK Mehta and Dr Haldipurkar Suhas who were pioneers in phaco surgery in India.

In 2002, I was with Padmashri Professor Dr TP Lahane, to attend European Society of Cataract and Refractive Surgeons (ESCRS) at Nice, France. After seeing this man, I was recharged in my ophthalmic career both academic and nonacademic way. I used to discuss points concerned with phaco surgery with him and Dr Ragini Parekh of JJ Hospital, Mumbai, Maharashtra.

In 2002, I started phaco training course. It was my passion to start such course. It was my habit to share the views with my colleagues. Since 2002, many doctors visited Navneet Hospital, Solapur from India and different parts of the world. Everyday discussions, analysis on the steps of phaco surgery with doctors, gave new ideas related to subject. In this course every day I used to learn new things out of discussion with colleagues. All these views, ideas and concepts related to phaco, I gathered in the form of notes.

I have tried to put all these notes in a concise way to prepare this book on phaco. This book is nothing, but my personal notes. It is concerned mainly with technical details and experienced views related to phaco.

Navneet Toshniwal

Acknowledgments

Blessings of the late Dr Sham Toshniwal and my mother, Chand Toshniwal are the most important part of my life to do this noble work of teaching. I express my heartfelt gratitude towards all my Toshniwal family members, especially Dr Nikhil, Dr Ayushi, and Dr Sumit, who have taken a lot of efforts to help me edit this book. Thanks to Dr Amit, Dr Abhishek, and Dr Nandini—the next generation of doctors of our family. Special efforts and support by my wife Sunita to complete this book. Thanks to Dr Nitin, Dr Neeta, Dr Kirti, and Dr Nilesh for encouraging me to write this book. My thanks to Dr Ashit Mehta and Sanjay Dargad for their kind help. Thanks to my colleagues, Dr Dilip Shirsikar, Dr Nitin Shah, and Dr S Jayram for their guidance.

I am also grateful to Shri Jitendar P Vij (Group Chairman), Mr Ankit Vij (Managing Director), Ms Chetna Malhotra (Senior Director—Professional Publishing, Marketing, and Business Development), and Ms Nikita Chauhan (Publishing Manager) of M/s Jaypee Brothers Medical Publishers (P) Ltd, New Delhi, India, who encouraged me to write this new edition.

I receive great motivation and encouragement from all my trainee doctors and fellows, who always insist me to come up with the 2nd edition of this very useful book.

Contents

1. Anatomy and Development of Lens 1
2. Selection of Patient 6
3. Phacoemulsification Machine... 19
4. Anesthesia 34
5. Bridle Sutures.. 38
6. Incision 41
7. Capsulorhexis.. 56
8. Hydroprocedures 75
9. Trench 80
10. Division of Nucleus 101
11. Hold and Chop of Nucleus.. 121
12. Removal of Small Pieces of Nucleus 145
13. Irrigation and Aspiration... 167
14. Intraocular Lens: Basic and Technical Aspects.............. 187
15. No Hydro in Phaco 193
16. Finishing Steps in Phacoemulsification Surgery 198
17. Instruments for Phaco Surgery 201

Index 209

Anatomy and Development of Lens

◾ INTRODUCTION

- The lens is a transparent, biconvex crystalline structure in the eye devoid of blood vessels and nerves that, along with the cornea, helps to refract light to be focused on the retina.
- The lens, by changing shape, functions toward changing the focal distance so that it can focus on objects at various distances, thus allowing a sharp real image of the object of interest to be formed on the retina.
- This adjustment of the lens is known as accommodation.
- In humans, the refractive power of the lens in its natural environment is approximately 18 diopters, roughly one third of the eye's total power.
- The lens is part of the anterior segment of the eye.
- Anterior to the lens is the iris which regulates the amount of light entering into the eye.
- The lens is suspended in place by the zonular fibers which are attached to the lens near its equatorial line and connect the lens to the ciliary body.
- Posterior to the lens is the vitreous body.
- The lens has an ellipsoid, biconvex shape. The anterior surface is less curved than the posterior.
- In adults, the lens is 10 mm in diameter and has an axial length of about 4–5 mm.
- **Figure 1** shows the anatomy of the lens.

◾ LENS CAPSULE

- The lens capsule is a smooth, transparent basement membrane that completely surrounds the lens.
- The capsule is elastic and composed of collagen.
- It is synthesized by the lens epithelium and its main components are type IV collagen and sulfated glycosaminoglycans (GAGs).

- As the capsule is very elastic, it causes the lens to assume a more globular shape when not under the tension of the zonular fibers, which connect the lens capsule to the ciliary body.
- The capsule varies from 4 to 20 µm in thickness, being the thickest near the equator and the thinnest near the posterior pole.
- The lens capsule may be involved with a higher anterior curvature than posterior of the lens.

■ LENS EPITHELIUM

- The lens epithelium is located in the anterior portion of the lens between the lens capsule and the lens fibers.
- It is a simple cuboidal epithelium.
- The cells of the lens epithelium regulate most of the homeostatic functions of the lens.
- The cells of the lens epithelium also serve as the progenitors for new lens fibers.
- The epithelium constantly lays down fibers in the embryo, fetus, infant, and adult, and continues to lay down fibers for lifelong growth.

■ LENS FIBERS

- The lens fibers form the bulk of the lens.
- They are long, thin, transparent cells firmly packed, with diameters between 4 and 8 µm and length up to 12 mm.
- The lens fibers stretch lengthwise from the posterior to the anterior poles and, when cut horizontally, are arranged in concentric layers.
- The middle of each fiber lies on the equator.
- These tightly packed layers of lens fibers are referred to as laminae.
- The lens fibers are linked together via gap junctions and interdigitations of the cells that resemble "ball and socket" forms.
- The lens is split into regions depending on the age of the lens fibers of a particular layer.
- Moving outward from the central, the oldest layer, the lens is split into an embryonic nucleus, the fetal nucleus, the adult nucleus, and the outer cortex.

- New lens fibers, generated from the lens epithelium, are added to the outer cortex. Mature lens fibers have no organelles or nuclei.

■ LENS PROTEINS
- These proteins are a class of crystallins.
- Crystallins are water-soluble proteins that compose over 90% of the protein within the lens.
- The three main crystallin types found in the human eye are α-, β-, and γ-crystallins.
- Crystallins tend to form soluble, high-molecular-weight aggregates that pack tightly in lens fibers; thus, it increases the index of refraction of the lens while maintaining its transparency.
- β- and γ-crystallins are found primarily in the lens, while subunits of α-crystallin have been isolated from other parts of the eye and the body.
- α-crystallin proteins mainly function to keep the lens transparent.
- Another important factor in maintaining the transparency of the lens is the absence of light-scattering cellular organelles.
- Lens fibers also have a very extensive cytoskeleton that maintains the precise shape and packing of the lens fibers.
- Disruptions of certain cytoskeleton elements can lead to the loss of transparency.

■ LENS METABOLISM
- The lens is metabolically active.
- Compared to other tissues in the eye, however, the lens has less energy demand.
- *Metabolism is by:*
  - Glycolysis (80%)
  - Hexose monophosphate shunt (18%)
  - Krebs cycle (1–2%)
- The lens receives all of its nourishment from the aqueous humor.
- Nutrients diffuse in and waste diffuses out through a constant flow of fluid from the anterior/posterior poles of the lens and out of the equatorial regions.
- Glucose is the primary energy source for the lens.

■ DEVELOPMENT OF LENS

- Development of the human lens begins at 4 mm embryonic stage.
- The lens is derived from the surface ectoderm.
- The first stage of lens differentiation takes place when the optic vesicle, which is formed from outpocketing in the neural ectoderm, comes in proximity to the surface ectoderm.
- The optic vesicle induces nearby surface ectoderm to form the lens placode.
- At 4 mm stage, the lens placode is a single monolayer of columnar cells.
- As development progresses, the lens placode begins to deepen and invaginate. As the placode continues to deepen, the opening to the surface ectoderm constricts and the lens cells form a structure known as the lens vesicle.
- By 10 mm stage, the lens vesicle is completely separated from the surface ectoderm.
- After the 10 mm stage, signals from the developing neural retina induce the cells closest to the posterior end of the lens vesicle and begin to elongate toward the anterior end of the vesicle.
- These signals also induce the synthesis of crystallins. These elongating cells eventually fill in the lumen of the vesicle to form the primary fibers, which become the embryonic nucleus in the mature lens.
- The cells of the anterior portion of the lens vesicle give rise to lens epithelium.
- Additional secondary fibers are derived from lens epithelial cells located toward the equatorial region of the lens.
- These cells lengthen anteriorly and posteriorly to encircle the primary fibers. The new fibers grow longer than those of the primary layer, but as the lens gets larger, the ends of the new fibers cannot reach the posterior or anterior poles of the lens. The lens fibers that do not reach the poles form tight, interdigitating seams with neighboring fibers. These seams are readily visible and are termed sutures. The suture patterns become more complex as more layers of lens fibers are added to the outer portion of the lens.

Anatomy and Development of Lens

- The lens continues to grow after birth, with the new secondary fibers being added as outer layers. New lens fibers are generated from the equatorial cells of the lens epithelium in a region referred to as the germinative zone. The lens epithelial cells elongate, lose contact with the capsule and epithelium, synthesize crystallin, and then finally lose their nuclei as they become mature lens fibers.
- From development through early adulthood, the addition of secondary lens fibers results in the lens growing more ellipsoid in shape; after about the age of 20 years, however, the lens grows more round with time.

■ KEY POINT

Put the picture of anatomy of lens in operation theater in first few days of phaco practice.

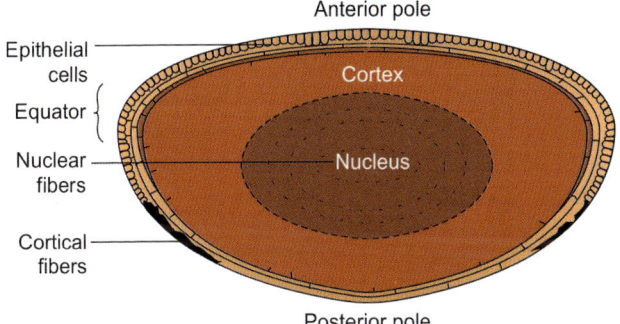

Fig. 1: Anatomy of lens.

CHAPTER 2

Selection of Patient

■ INTRODUCTION

Selection of the patient is the most important and crucial part for the success in phaco surgery. **Figures 1 to 12** show the different cataracts and possible phaco surgery to manage it.

■ HISTORY

As with other surgeries, taking history is very important. History includes the history of patient, family history, systemic disease especially of diabetes mellitus, hypertension, ischemic heart disease, asthma, previous ocular surgeries, and taking systemic and local medication.

■ GENERAL EXAMINATION

Age of Patient

In author's opinion, age is the most important factor for surgery that one should not take casually. Aging means more degeneration. As the age advances, the anatomy of the lens shows some changes such as zonular weakness and thinning of anterior and posterior capsules; it means that the overall bag in which the surgery is performed may be weak. More age means harder nucleus; more age means size of nucleus is big. In author's opinion, size of nucleus is more significant than hardness.

Texture of Body

Kyphosis, scoliosis, parkinsonism, tremors, weight of patient, and paralytic patient.

Patient's Ability of Hearing

It is very important to take cooperation of the patient during surgery.

Language of Patient

Ability to understand language of patient is important for primary steps of surgery like during anesthesia and during bridle sutures, incision, and capsulorhexis.

Cooperation of Patient

Cooperation of patient may be very important for any surgery.

Mental Intellect of Patient

Surgeons can do topical phaco surgery.

■ SYSTEMIC EXAMINATION

Hypertension and Ischemic Heart Disease

One should see hypertensive retinopathy changes and drugs used for it. Usually, you have to stop anticoagulants before surgery.

Diabetes Mellitus

See for diabetic retinopathy. Most important factor for diabetes mellitus is diabetic cataract. Types of cataract in diabetics are:
- Soft cataract
- Hard, brown cataract
- Hydrated lens
- *Mature cataract:* Hard or soft
- Sticky cataract
- Leathery texture cataract
- Posterior subcapsular cataract
- Cataract in young age
- Cataract in old age
- Anterior subcapsular cataract

Asthmatic: These patients are usually on steroid, so steroid-induced posterior subcapsular cataract is seen. Positive pressure during surgery can occur.

Allergy to drugs: History of allergy of drugs either systemic or local eye drops (e.g., mydriatic eye drops containing phenylephrine and atropine).

Current consumption of medication: Medication for systemic illnesses such as hypertension, diabetes mellitus, and asthma and any medication for other systemic diseases should be continued before and after surgery.

Medicine such as aspirin and other anticoagulants should be discontinued 2–3 days prior to surgery.

■ OTHER FACTORS

Occupational History

Working atmosphere of patient, such as in factories where heat-induced and radiation-induced cataracts are prevalent. Radiation-induced cataract is seen in X-ray technicians and radiologists.

History of Trauma

Cataract varies from case to case.

■ LOCAL EXAMINATION

Examination under torch light and slit-lamp examination.

Position of Eyeball

This is done to see deep socket. Superior and inferior rectus bridle sutures are very important in these cases. In superior approach, clear corneal incision may be the preferred incision over the limbal incision, as the working space is less. Also, the type of phaco tip preferred in such situation is the Kelman tip. Temporal approach may be preferred to a superior approach.

Palpebral Fissure

In narrow palpebral fissure, there is difficulty for the superior approach of surgery and superior rectus and inferior rectus bridle sutures are necessary in such cases. Temporal incision may be the preferred incision in such cases.

Eyelids

One should look for signs suggestive of meibomitis as the oily secretion may hamper the visualization during surgery and here one needs to wash the conjunctival sac continuously with balanced salt solution and cotton buds.

Conjunctiva and Sclera

One should look for conjunctival thinning or inflammation and also for scleral thinning and inflammation and caution should be taken during surgery. Also, one should look for signs of old surgeries such as bleb of glaucoma surgery, buckles of retinal surgery, post pterygium cases and accordingly modify the incision and further steps of surgery.

Cornea

Here, one should look for corneal opacity and haziness, as a clear cornea is required for visualization during surgery. Associated pterygium and also other factors affecting the astigmatism should be considered when concern is about preoperative and postoperative astigmatism of the patient. Nowadays, keratometry (manual and automated) topography and pachymetry are important to select the site of incision during surgery and also to do limbal relaxing incisions (LRIs) to correct corneal astigmatism postsurgical. It is very important for toric lenses also.

Anterior Chamber Depth

It is the most important factor among all the factors in the author's opinion. A normal anterior chamber depth is one of the crucial factors for successful phaco surgery.

Shallow Anterior Chamber

Relatively shallow anterior chamber depth is important to notice preoperatively as the working space of the surgery is reduced. Also, the probes are near to cornea, anterior capsule, posterior capsule, and iris and so chances of complication are more and also the workup needs to be done in a compact space. One must always see the associated findings with shallow anterior chamber depth, such as small pupil, pseudoexfoliation, hypermetropia, and convex anterior capsule. In shallow anterior chamber depth, the speed and movement of surgery is slow (slow motion surgery). Putting visco in shallow anterior chamber depth is an art and always considers the volume of anterior chamber to that of visco which put in anterior chamber. In shallow anterior chamber depth, the chances of iris prolapse are very common via any port and so the architecture of incision size and valvular effect of all the ports should be perfect. In shallow anterior chamber depth, the main port and side ports should be sufficiently away from each other and side port should be clear corneal. Capsulorhexis is more difficult in shallow anterior chamber depth, and one should always try to make a small rhexis. Passing all the instruments to the anterior chamber is also difficult. Consideration of anatomy is important for case selection as for shallow anterior chamber with soft nucleus, one can try phaco surgery, but for shallow anterior chamber with hard nucleus, one should think about other surgical options.

Deep Anterior Chamber

Deep anterior chamber is usually safe for cornea but is fearsome and can be associated with subluxated lens, myopia, hypotony, etc.

Examination of Pupil

Examination of pupil in pre- and postdilatation is important. Size and shape of pupil should be marked on indoor paper; if it is eccentric, then one has to make the size and shape of the pupil toward the center by sphincterotomy, which is called pupilloplasty. Adequately dilated pupils are prerequisite for good phaco surgery. A mid-dilated pupil after installing mydriatic drops is suggestive that the pupils can become small intraoperatively. Anterior chamber depth is always assessed perfectly in undilated pupil. Pupil of the other eye is helpful to assess the size and shape of the pupil in the operative eye. In postoperative cases, if pupil is central and round, it increases the confidence of the operating surgeon for other eye.

If there is updrawn pupil postoperatively in first eye, one should be careful while operating the other eye.

Lens

- Torchlight examination will give an idea about the hardness of the lens by seeing the color. It also gives an idea about the maturity of nucleus.
- Slit-lamp examination is the most important tool for the selection of the patients for cataract surgery. Apart from examination of other structures, the anatomy of the lens should be seen in detail post dilatation. Grading of the nucleus is also done in slit-lamp examination. This gives an idea about the hardness of the nucleus.

Grading of Nucleus (Hardness)

- Color
  - *Grade 1:* Mild yellow
  - *Grade 2:* Yellow
  - *Grade 3:* Yellowish-brown
  - *Grade 4:* Brown
  - *Grade 5:* Dark-brown or black

Size of the Nucleus

This is one of the most neglected parts of examination of the nucleus and is very important for selection of cases for successful cataract surgery. Study of correlation of the size of nucleus with the dilated pupil size has very rewarded results in the successful phaco practice.

Examination of Lens in Detail

- Zonular integrity and strength should be noticed overall.
- Site of lenticular opacity varies from case to case and surgery can be modified accordingly.
- *Classification depending upon the site of opacity can be:*
  - Anterior capsular, anterior subcapsular, or posterior subcapsular cataract
  - Nuclear cataract

Selection of Patient

- Posterior polar cataract
- Cortical cataract
- Mature cataract

- Weak zones in the lens can be seen after dilation of both the eyes. These are usually seen as abnormal shadows in the lens, especially seen in retro illumination.
- All the layers of the nucleus should be visible during slit examination of slit-lamp examination. This is usually not possible in hard nucleus sclerosis IV or mature cataract; in such situations, it is usually an unpredictable surgery.
- Grading of the nucleus can also be done under indirect ophthalmoscopy—this is done to detect the central hardness of nucleus. If the posterior pole of fundus is seen clearly on examination, then the hardness is less; with increase in the hardness of nucleus, the visualization becomes less and in cases of no visualization, one must reconsider the option of a phaco surgery or convert to small-incision cataract surgery or extracapsular cataract surgery.

Both eye examinations: Ophthalmologists are very lucky as they can compare one eye anatomy with that of the other.
- Corneal haziness in one eye is considered as weak cornea in normal eye also.
- Anterior chamber depth can also be assessed in other eye.
- Pseudoexfoliation in one eye suggests weak zonules may be in the other eye.
- In mature cataract, the examination of the other eye gives an idea about suspected hidden abnormality of anatomy of lens in the selected eye.
- Coloboma of the iris gives the idea about weak zonules in the other eye.
- Subluxated lens in one eye is suggestive of weak zonules in the other eye too.

Examination in lying down position: It gives an idea about position of the eyeball prior to surgery, the anterior chamber depth assessment, and hidden subluxation of lens can be seen.

Selection of Patient 13

■ KEY POINT
Selection and analysis of presumption of steps of phaco surgery by doing slit-lamp examination before surgery is the most important factor for successful and safe surgery.

▍ SLIT-LAMP PHOTOGRAPHS OF CATARACT— SELECTION AND ANALYSIS (FIGS. 1 TO 12)

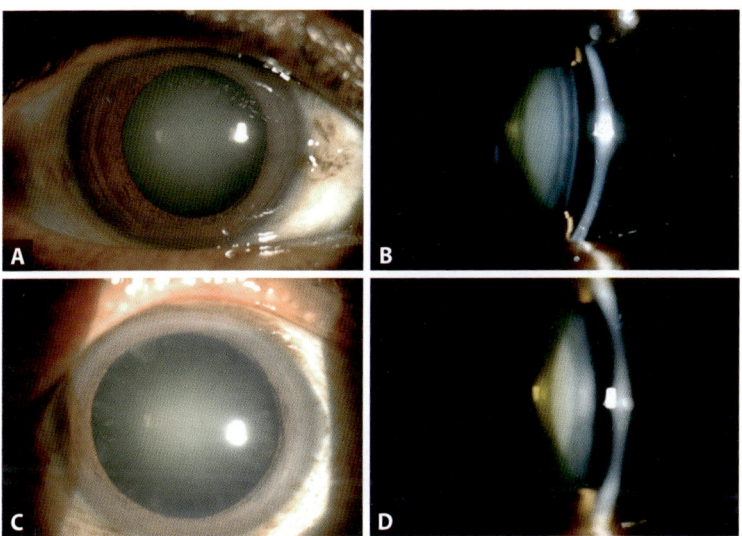

Figs. 1A to D: Grade II nucleus—all layers of lens can be seen (ideal case).

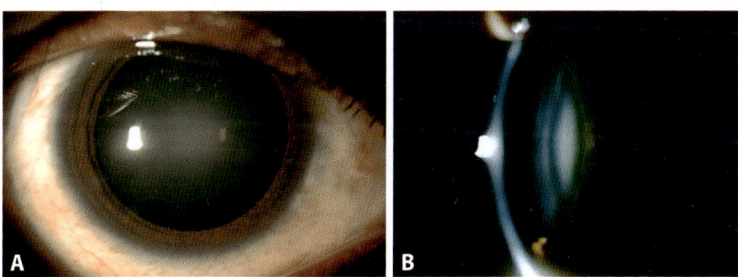

Figs. 2A and B: Phaco in small nucleus. Different ways to manage small nucleus—not very difficult.

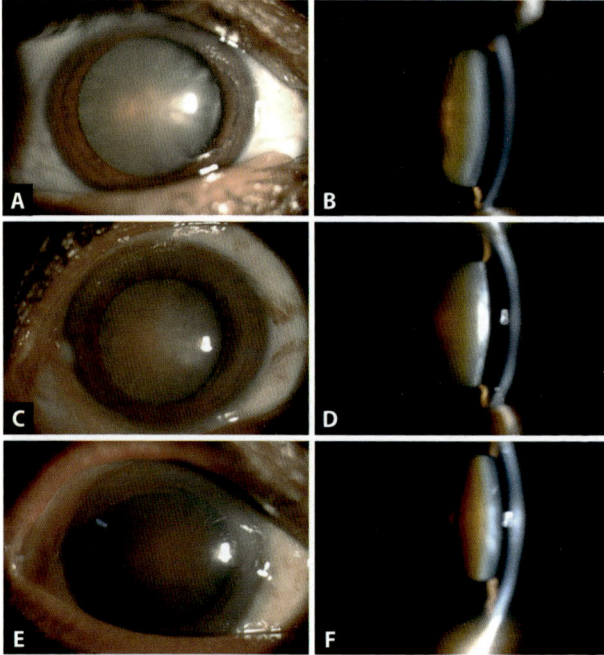

Figs. 3A to F: Hard cataract with different hardness of nucleus and different sizes of nucleus.

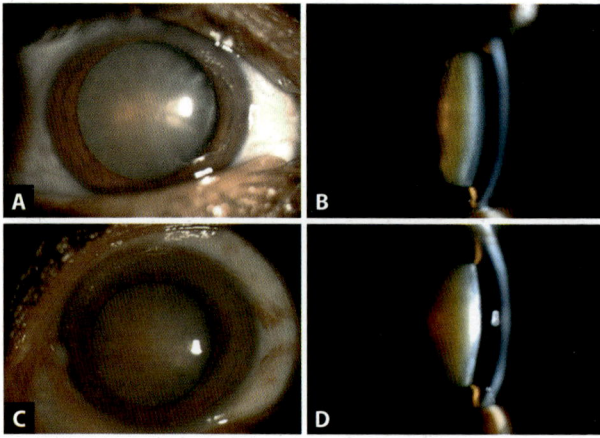

Figs. 4A to D: (A and B) Hard cataract—big-size nucleus. One can see layers of anatomy, anterior and posterior demarcation can be seen, so predictable phaco; (C and D) Big-size nucleus—layer of nucleus not defined, so difficult and unpredictable to do phaco.

Selection of Patient

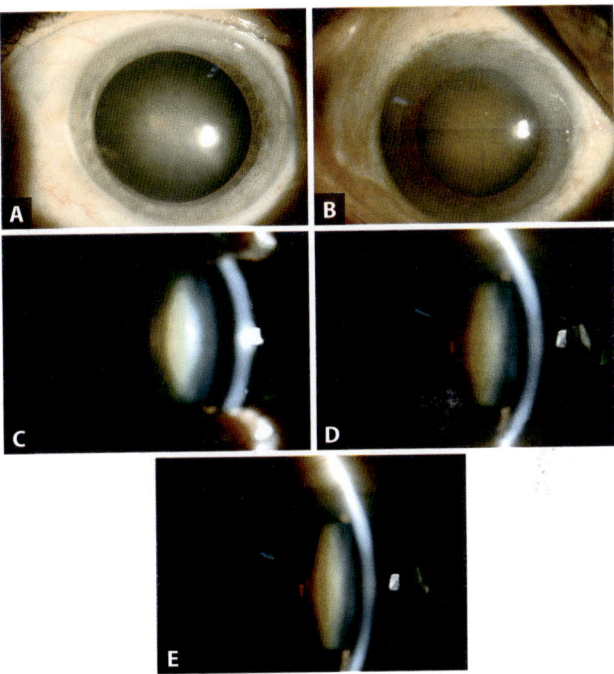

Figs. 5A to E: Hard with small-size nucleus, comparatively easy to do phaco (ideal case).

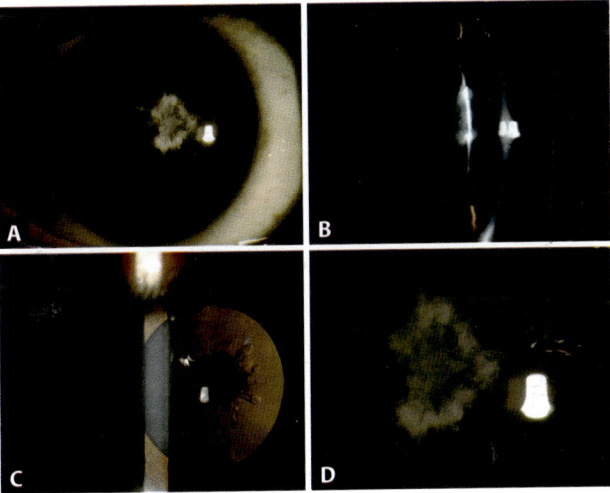

Figs. 6A to D: Anterior subcapsular cataract (difficult to do rhexis).

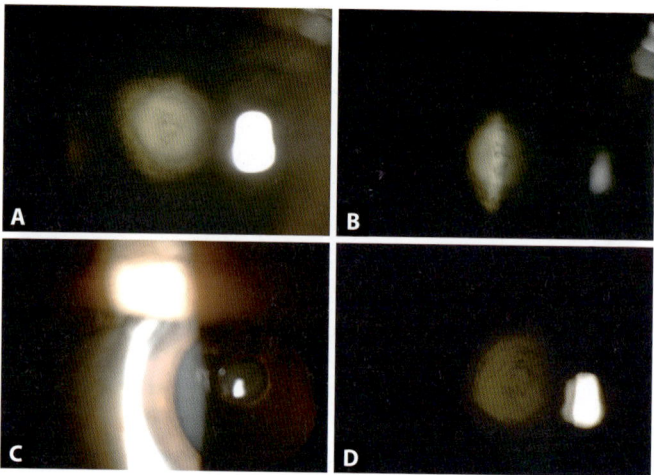

Figs. 7A to D: Posterior polar cataract (challenge for a cataract surgeon by any technique).

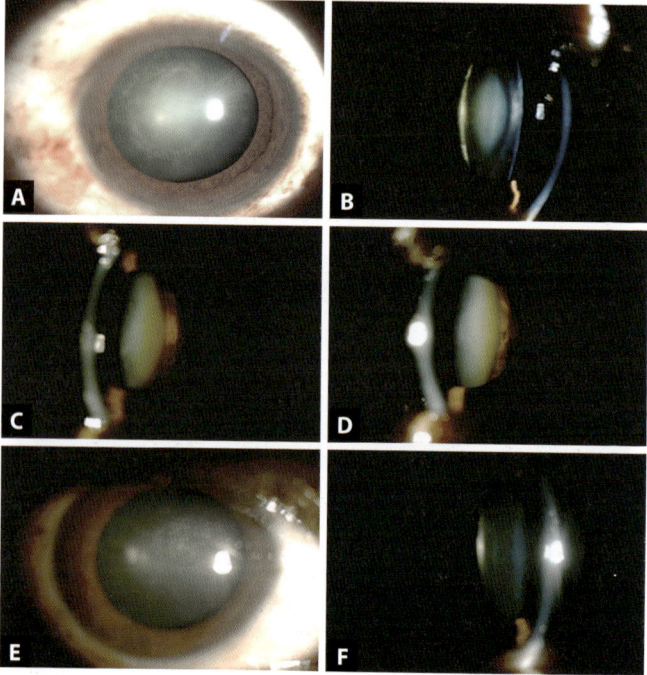

Figs. 8A to F: Posterior subcapsular cataract: (A and B) Good case, good nucleus size; (C and D) Big-size nucleus, so difficult or unpredictable phaco; and (E and F) No nucleus, so difficult or unpredictable phaco.

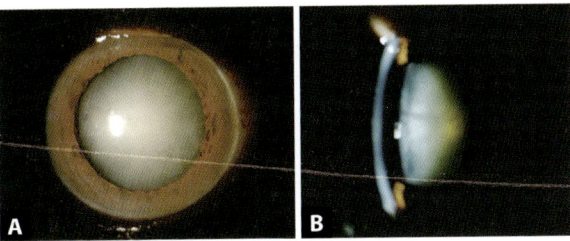

Figs. 9A and B: Cortical cataract with big-size nucleus and soft nucleus—irrigation aspiration is difficult.

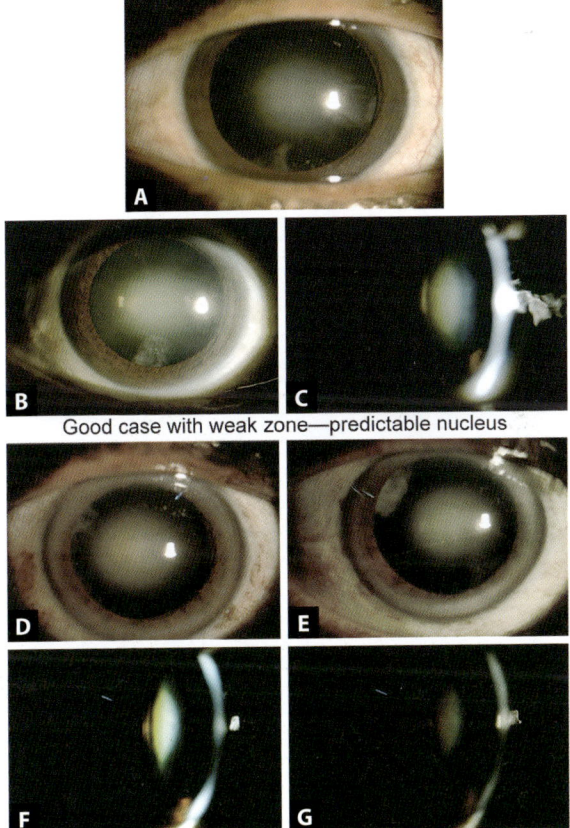

Good case with weak zone—predictable nucleus

Good case I/A—difficult in that weak zone

Figs. 10A to G: Cataract with weak zone: (A) Weak zone and (B to G) weak zone with adequate-size nucleus—predictable phaco, but irrigation aspiration is difficult in that weak zone.

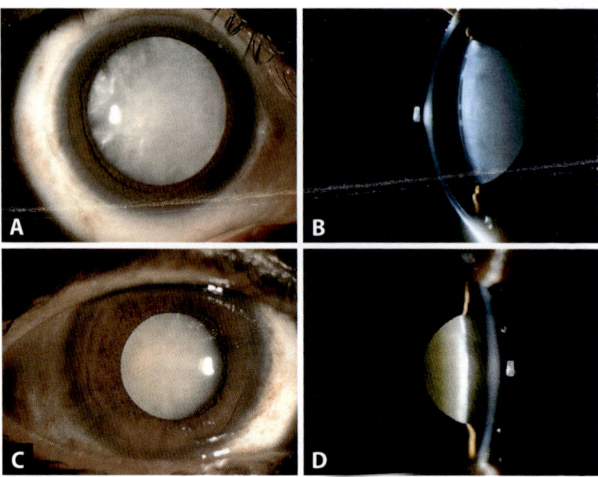

Figs. 11A to D: Mature cataract—layer of nucleus cannot be differentiated so unpredictable phaco.

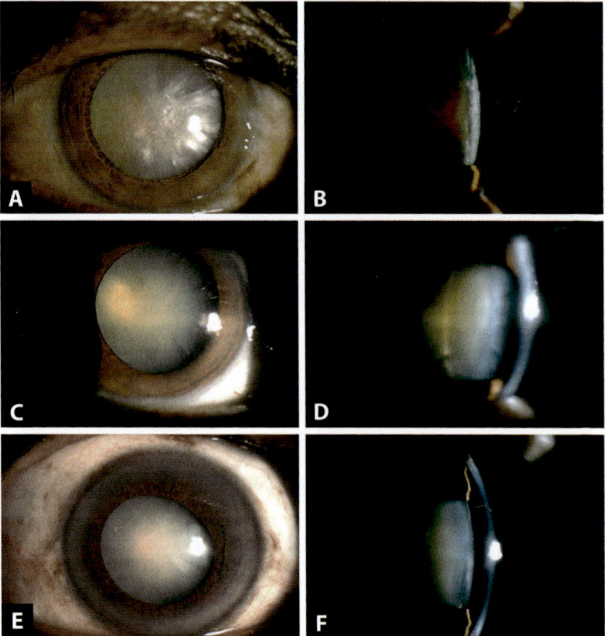

Figs. 12A to F: Mature cataract for phaco. Always unpredictable but still can think of phaco as—can differentiate layers of cataract and can know size and hardness of nucleus before start of surgery on slit-lamp.

CHAPTER 3

Phacoemulsification Machine

■ INTRODUCTION

Phaco surgery is a machine-dependent surgery to understand that the basic functioning of the phaco machine is integral part for success of phaco surgery. Simplicity of phaco surgery depends upon how one knows the machines thoroughly. Complication rate is reduced with good knowledge of surgeon's own phaco machine. One should give sufficient time to get accustomed and to customize the parameters related to steps of phaco surgery.

■ PARTS OF PHACO MACHINE

Console (Figs. 1 and 2)

It contains basic hardware and software of the machine. On the display screen, all the parameters are shown such as energy, vacuum, and aspiration and irrigation flow rates and their details.

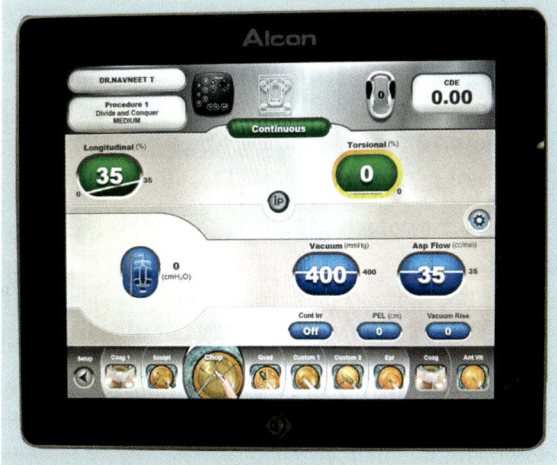

Fig. 1: Console of ALCON legion machine.

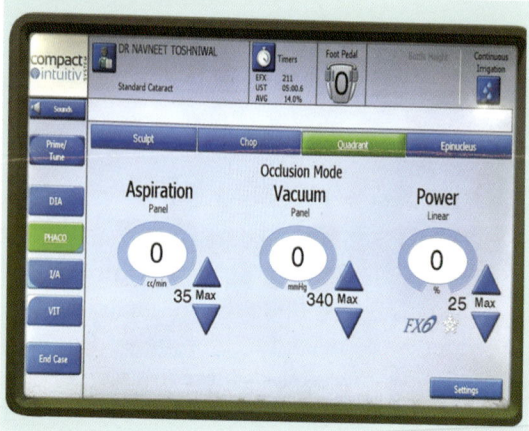

Fig. 2: Console of Intuitiv machine.

Pumps

Three types of pumps are present:
1. Venturi pump
2. Diaphragmatic pump
3. Peristaltic pump

Venturi Pump

There is no discrimination between vacuum and aspiration flow rate, which means that both are working together.

Principle: Compressed gas creates a negative suction force that is the vacuum inside a closed chamber which is directly transmitted to the handpiece.

Advantages:
- Surgical procedure is fast.
- Vacuum works more efficiently and thus, holding capacity of the machine for the nucleus is better.

Disadvantages:
- Being a fast machine, the safety zone is less.
- Catching of iris and iris chaffing
- Catching of anterior and posterior capsule is common.

Diaphragmatic Pump

A diaphragm pump is having flexible membrane to generate vacuum. With this pump, vacuum reaches to preset level without occlusion. This mechanism is easy to remove small pieces, but safety margin is less.

Peristaltic Pump

It is one of the most widely used pump in the practice of phaco. Vacuum and aspiration flow rate work independently but finally assisting each other.

Principle: In peristaltic pump, the rotation of the rollers by the pump pinches the soft silicon tubing, which creates a negative pressure by squeezing the fluid out of the tube. In this system, the vacuum will be built up only when the tip is occluded.

Advantages:
- Safe machine
- No fear at any level of surgical skill of the surgeon
- Complicated cases can be handled safely and in a skillful way
- Level of confidence of workup is maintained throughout the procedure
- Chances of catching of iris, capsule is less.

Disadvantages:
- According to some surgeon's point of view, it is a slow machine.
- In some machines, both the peristaltic and venturi pumps work together.

Tubing (Figs. 3A and B)

Phaco machine attaches to the phaco probe via this tubing. Two functions of the tubing are irrigation and aspiration. These tubings are made up of silicon material which can be autoclaved or ethylene oxide (ETO) sterilized. With the higher-end machines, one can get presterile pouch of tubing which is called cassette. Phaco fluidics depend upon the quality of tubing.

Factors determining the quality of reusable tubing are:
- *Color:* Yellow color indicates an old tubing which should ideally be changed.

Phacoemulsification Machine

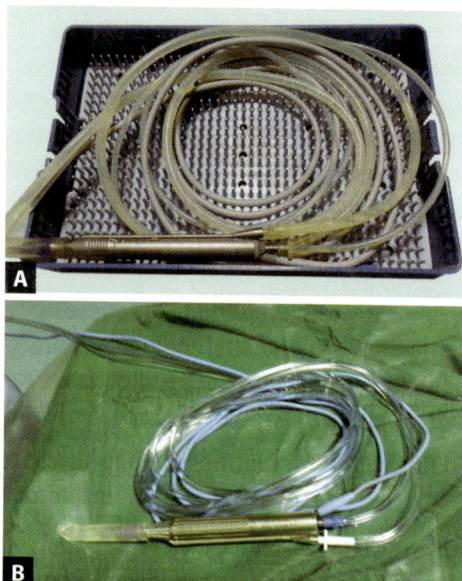

Figs. 3A and B: Tubing of phaco machine.

- *Consistency of the tubing:* Hard consistency of tubing which is not flexible should be changed.
- *Fitting:* Ends of the tubing which are attached to the machine and the phaco probe should not be loose.
- If the ends of the tubing are not smooth or appear damaged, then the tubing should be changed.

Cassette—in higher-end machines, disposable cassettes are used.

Phaco Probe

It is a piezoelectric substance which converts electronic energy to mechanical energy, and thus giving the ultrasound energy under the influence of electrical signal.

Frequency: 30,000–60,000 Hz (commonly used are 40,000 Hz). Different probes have different number of crystals ranging from 2 to 4. More the crystal, more is the stroke length and more is the power.

Parts

- Phaco handpiece **(Figs. 4A and B)**
- *Phaco tip:* Hollow titanium tip **(Figs. 5A and B)**
- *Wrench:* Phaco tip is screwed into the handpiece by wrench **(Fig. 6)**.

Function of the probe is to deliver the energy that emulsifies the hard part of cataract which is the nucleus.

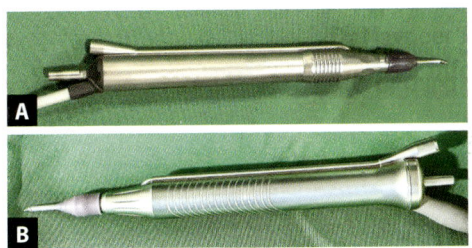

Figs. 4A and B: Phaco handpiece.

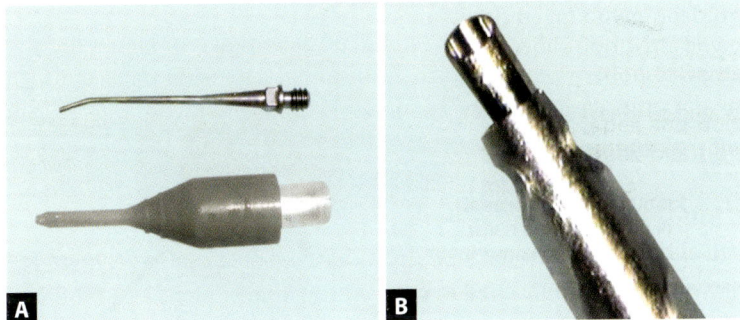

Figs. 5A and B: Phaco tip.

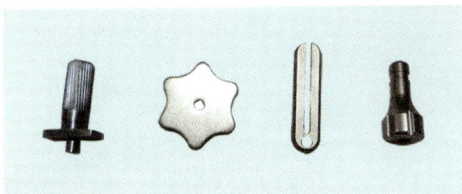

Fig. 6: Wrench.

The mechanism of working is by:
- *Jackhammer effect:* It is the direct mechanical impact on the nucleus to emulsify it.
- *Cavitational effect:* Between the phaco tip and the nucleus, the bubbles form in irrigating fluid in this gap which emulsify the tissue.
- *Acoustic wave of fluid:* This is generated by the forward movement of the tip, which can disintegrate the lens material.

Power of the machine depends upon the stroke length and the frequency remains fixed.

Methods to check an ideal phaco handpiece:
- Weight of the phaco probe should not be very heavy.
- Length of the probe should not be too long or small.
- Grip on probe should be perfect.
- It should be friendly in use; this means moving down, up, and sideways should be free.
- There should be no kinking of the tubing at the proximal end of the phaco probe.

Holding of a phaco probe should be like a pen grip. Generally, the angulation between the phaco probe and the incision ranges from 0° to 30°, otherwise there are chances of damage to the architecture of the incision.

Phaco Tips (Figs. 7 and 8)

There are different varieties of tips used in practice. These are straight tip, Kelman tip, flared tip, Turbosonics microtip, and flared aspiration bypass system (ABS) tip.

There are two tips available in the market, the 19-gauge tip and 20-gauge tip.

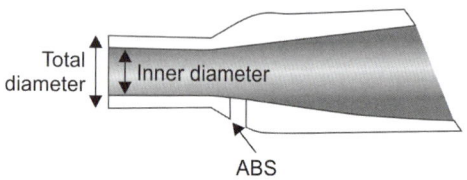

Fig. 7: Design of flared aspiration of bypass system (ABS) phaco tip.

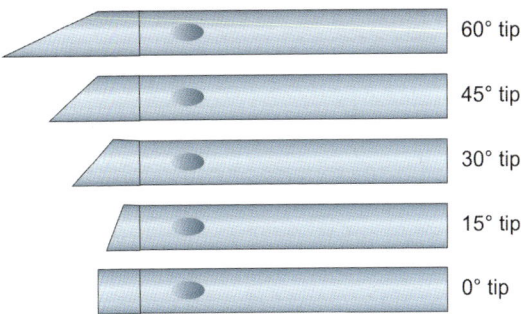

Fig. 8: Phaco tip with different angulations.

Cutting efficiency is better with the 45° tip (effect) and hold is better with 0° tip (effect).

Sleeve (Fig. 9)

Sleeve is made of silicon material which covers the phaco tip. It protects the cornea and iris from transmitted heat energy by the probe. The fluid for the irrigation flows between the sleeve and phaco tip, thus cooling the tip. There are two openings 180° apart on the sleeve through which irrigating fluid exits the sleeve. The size of the incision depends upon tip gauge and the sleeve. The gauge of the phaco tip is fixed, but if you want to pass the phaco tip from 1.8 to 2.8 mm incision, it depends upon the thickness of the sleeve. Many companies come with different color codes for the various thicknesses of sleeves.

The distance between the distal end of the phaco tip and that of the sleeve (exposed part of the phaco tip) defers from case to case. Hard cataract may need more exposed part of the tip and a softer cataract may need a small exposed part of the tip.

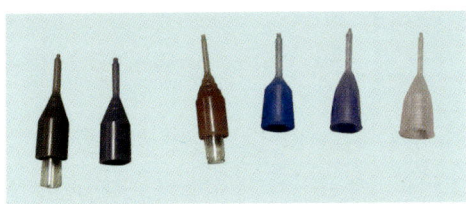

Fig. 9: Different types of sleeves.

Direction of irrigation fluid flow depends upon the placement of the sleeve over the phaco tip and this finally plays a very important role in phaco fluidics.

Sleeve is autoclaved or ETO sterilized.

A sleeve should be changed when:
- Elasticity is altered and it becomes loosely fit over the phaco tip.
- There is difficulty while going through incision.
- Sleeve gets torn or there is a hole in the sleeve.
- Discoloration of the sleeve occurs.

Test Chamber (Fig. 10)

- It is again silicon made and is helpful for tuning of the machine and before start of the case, it is useful to have an idea about the parameters of the machine in the test chamber with balanced salt solution (BSS).
- If a small nucleus particle is stuck in the tip or aspiration port of tubing, it can be removed in the test chamber with BSS solution in the energy mode of the machine.
- Sometimes, it is also used for research purpose to see the behavior of nucleus pieces in various modes of energy.
- Test chamber gives protection to the phaco tip.

When to change the test chamber:
- If it is torn or there is a hole
- Discoloration of the test chamber

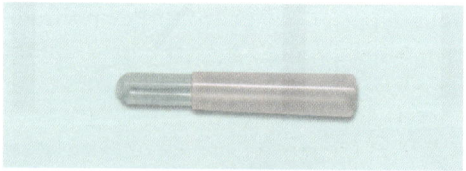

Fig. 10: Test chamber.

Foot Pedal (Figs. 11 and 12)

Learning the use of foot pedal is like learning the accelerator of the car. This is one of the most important aspects in phaco surgery that one should learn the control of foot pedal.

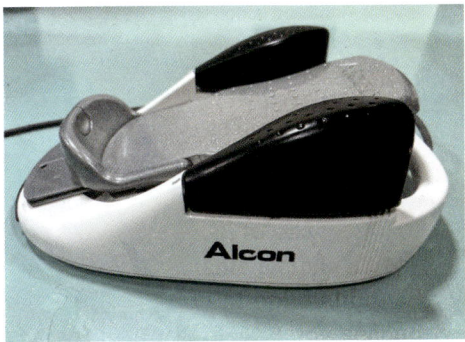

Fig. 11: Foot pedal side view.

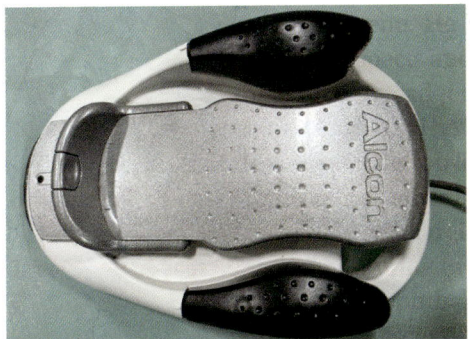

Fig. 12: Foot pedal front view.

There are three positions of foot pedal **(Fig. 13)**. A surgeon presses foot pedal down in the following order:
1. A: Position one—irrigation
2. A + B: Position two—irrigation and aspiration
3. A + B + C: Position three—irrigation, aspiration, and energy

There are gaps among these three settings that are present and can be preset by the machine which can be varied according to the surgeons. There are audible and tactile sensations to detect the position of foot pedal. The foot pedal position should be comfortable to the surgeon.

In some machines, all the parameters can be controlled by *foot pedal*.

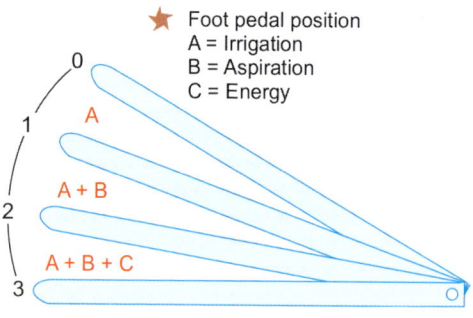

Fig. 13: Foot pedal position.

Reflux: All foot pedals have a unique control called reflux control. The basic principle is repulsion of the fluid and aspirated material like posterior capsule or iris that has been accidentally caught in the aspiration port.

PREPARATION OR TUNING OF THE PHACO MACHINE

This is the first important step before phaco surgery. Various machines have different ways to do this step. Most important step is connecting the irrigation aspiration tubing for the tuning of the machine.

CLEANING OF PHACO MACHINE

It varies from machine to machine. Basic principle is to remove nucleus material and debris out of the aspiration port of tubing. After cleaning, the machine tubing should be dry before sterilization.

Both tuning and cleaning of machine can be learned from technicians of company.

IMPORTANT TERMS CONCERNED WITH THE PHACO MACHINE

Linear

This means a gradual rise in the values of the mode to the preset level from zero with linear relation to the foot pedal control.

Panel

Sudden increase or rise in the values from zero to the preset value as soon as the foot pedal is pressed.

Energy

It is the ultrasound energy. Simple definition of energy is the ability to emulsify the tissue, mainly the nucleus mass. It depends upon stroke length, frequency, and efficiency of phaco probe.

Stroke Length

It is the distance by which phaco tip moves to and fro. It can be altered by changing the phaco power. It means that more the phaco power, more is the stroke length, more is the distance of cut made ahead of the phaco tip.

Frequency

It is the number of times the tip moves and is fixed for every phaco handpiece. It is measured in kHz.

Different Modes of Energy (Fig. 14)

Continuous Energy

This is the energy without any gap. It is used for trench and during the hold to engage the nucleus.

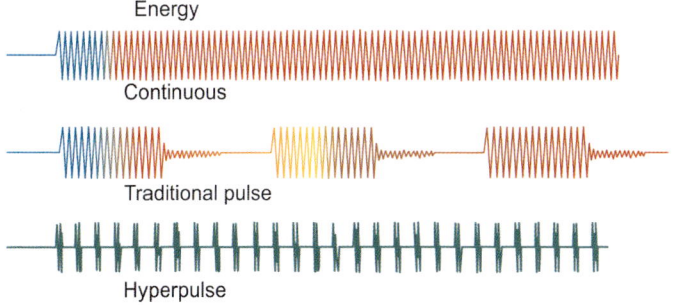

Fig. 14: Different modes of energy.

Traditional Pulse Energy

Adequate energy followed by minimum energy followed by no energy and again adequate energy- minimum energy- no energy and the cycle continues. It is used for the controlled removal of small pieces after the chop. Sometimes, it is also used to engage the nucleus for hold. It is never used for trench.

Hyperpulse Energy

Hyperpulse energy is also called *microburst* or *whitestar energy (cold phaco)*—this is widely used form of energy. It can be used for:
- Trench
- To engage the nucleus for hold
- Emulsifying of small pieces
  All depends on on and off time of duty cycle.
  1 second is equal to 1,000 ms and there are different formulae C/F or B/D.

Advantages of hyperpulse:
- Energy delivered is very less.
- Magnetic followability of the tissue is seen.

Burst Mode

It is like panel mode where energy is fixed and frequency of phaco bursts will increase with pressing the foot pedal more and more. It means that one burst per second to start with and then with full pressing of foot pedal, energy is continuous.

Torsional Energy

Torsional energy works with Kelman tip only and machine used is Legion and Centurion. Here, emulsification of nucleus is done by shearing forces. Most important advantage is that there is no repulsion of pieces, better cutting efficiency, and minimal surge. Surgeons can get all advantages of Kelman tip.

Vacuum

It is the ability of holding the tissue. It is in mm of mercury. It is the difference in pressure between the atmospheric pressure and the pressure inside the tubing. This is a negative suction pressure created by the pumps.

Aspiration Flow Rate

It is the amount of fluid coming out of the eye in cc per minute. In simple words, it denotes followability of the tissue.

Rise Time

The rise time is time taken by machine to reach maximum preset vacuum after occlusion has been achieved.

Surge

Sudden release of the occlusion of the phaco tip leads to sudden gush of fluid from the anterior chamber to the phaco tip, leading to sudden collapse of anterior chamber. This is called surge. In other words, sudden collapse of anterior chamber due to withdrawal of fluid from the anterior chamber to the tip after occlusion breaks is called surge.

Mechanism of surge (**Fig. 15**): During the removal of nucleus pieces when piece is away from the phaco tip, the rollers are rotating, no occlusion or collapse of tubing occurs, but when occlusion of the tip with the nucleus pieces occurs, vacuum builds up, pumps stop, and a negative pressure is generated within the system and so the tubing gets collapsed. After break of occlusion at one point, pressure is released and the tubing expands to the original size and fluid is

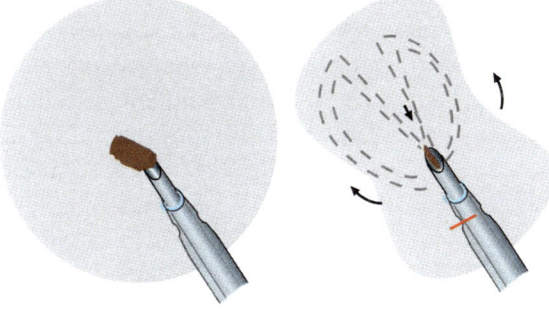

Fig. 15: Mechanism of surge.

drawn from the anterior chamber to fill up this extra volume of the tubing and so the chamber gets collapsed.

Complications due to surge:
- Posterior capsule rupture
- Iris trauma
- Endothelial damage

How to avoid surge:
- Increase the infusion fluid by:
  - Increasing the bottle height
  - Using the transurethral resection (TUR) set
  - Additional infusion by anterior chamber maintainer
- Decrease the parameters of machine like the aspiration flow rate and vacuum
- *Proper wound constructions:* There should not be leakage from the main or side port wound.
- *Foot pedal control is one of the most important aspects to avoid surge:* To move from foot position two to three and then back from three to two should be very well coordinated according to the step of surgery that is chopping or emulsifying of nucleus pieces.
- During the removal of small pieces or irrigation aspiration of epinucleus and cortex, the tip of phaco or irrigation aspiration port should be in opposition with the next mass before occlusion breaks.
- Some machines have sensor which detect occlusion break and avoid surge by release of fluid or air into the system.
- Some machines are having an option of different settings after the occlusion breaks. As soon as the occlusion breaks, the machine shifts its parameters (aspiration flow rate and vacuum) to the lower limit, thus preventing sudden gush of fluid from anterior chamber and thus prevents surge.

Chatter

When the energy used is more than adequate for the removal of small nucleus pieces, then repulsion of the nucleus piece away from the phaco tip occurs and this is called chatter.

Total ultrasound time: It is the total time during which the ultrasound energy is actually being delivered to emulsify the cataract.

Effective phaco time: It is calculated by the phaco machine. During the surgery, the surgeon uses various percentage of phaco energy from zero to preset for complete nucleus management (*actual phaco time*). Machine denotes that if surgeon uses its preset values all the time for nucleus management, it will take less duration than needed. This time calculated by the machine is called *effective phaco time*. For example, the machine takes 10 seconds with variable percentage of energy to emulsify nucleus, the same mass can be emulsified with continuous preset energy in 3 seconds. So actual phaco time is 10 seconds and effective phaco time is 3 seconds.

■ IRRIGATION AND ASPIRATION

- There is no parameter of energy.
- Same terminologies—linear and panel—are applicable.
- Details of this topic mentioned in further chapter of this book.
- Detail of all aspects of phaco machine is described in book 'Phaco machine and its application' written by author himself and published by M/s Jaypee Brothers Medical Publishers (P) Ltd.

■ KEY POINTS

- Learning phaco machine is like learning a car; therefore, it should be very slow and gradual for effective results.
- Spend some time with phaco machine to learn the details of machine.
- Maintenance of machine is important and usually, it should be handled by single person.
- Customization of parameter of our own phaco machine with our surgical steps are important.

Anesthesia

INTRODUCTION

- As in other surgical procedures, it plays a significant role in cataract surgery. It may be topical, local, or general anesthesia.
- Importance of anesthesia is that the patient should give good cooperation throughout the procedure without eye movements.
- Operative procedures should be painless.
- All the surgical steps are easy to do with good anesthesia.
- No fear of surgery for the patient.

TYPES OF ANESTHESIA

- Topical
- Local
- General

Local or Regional Anesthesia

- Anesthesia which is given near or around the eyeball
- *Different types of regional anesthesia:*
  - *Peribulbar anesthesia:*
    - Total 4–5 cc of xylocaine 2%, with or without adrenaline and senserocaine
      - First injection is given through lower eye lid at the junction of medial two-thirds and lateral one-third, either by pressing the eyeball up or by asking the patient to look straight or up. The needle is directed straight or slightly towards optic nerve. Before injecting, one should aspirate first to see if the needle is in the blood vessel or not. If blood comes during this maneuver, one should change the site either medially or laterally.
      - Second injection is given at junction of medial one-third and lateral two-thirds through the upper eyelid

by moving the eyeball down with fingers in straight direction.
- Usually, 3 cc is given via lower eyelid and 1 cc is given via upper eyelid.
- Quantity of anesthesia differs from patient to patient, and it depends upon the anatomy of the eye.
- *Facial and retrobulbar anesthesia:*
  - *O'Brian method:* 2–3 cc of mixture is given at the neck of mandible which is identified by asking the patient to open and close the mouth.
  - *Von Lint method:* 2–3 cc of the mixture is given at the bone margin lateral to lateral canthus. Half of the solution is directed toward the upper eyebrow and the other is directed opposite to it.
  - *Retrobulbar anesthesia:* 2–3 cc of the mixture is given at the junction of medial two-thirds and lateral one-third with 23-gauge needle with 1.5-inch length given through lower eye lid or at the same point by everting the lower eyelid and directed always toward the optic nerve in muscle cone.
- *Sub-Tenon's:*
  - 2–3 cc of xylocaine 2% is taken.
  - With the help of conjunctival scissors, conjunctival tenon incision is taken inferotemporally, 3 mm from limbus.
  - Sub-Tenon's canula is directed posteriorly and the solution is injected.
- *Subconjunctival anesthesia:* After taking the bridle sutures if pain persists, subconjunctival anesthesia of 0.2 cc is given by lifting the rectus.

Topical Anesthesia

- 4% xylocaine or 0.5% proparacaine hydrochloride is put two to three times, 15 minutes before surgery.
- 2% xylocaine jelly is instilled into the eye 10 minutes before surgery by some surgeons.

General Anesthesia

- It is given by anesthesiologists with their own techniques.

- It has three phases:
  1. *Induction phase:*
     - This can be done with propofol or ketamine.
     - These are fast-acting and short-duration type of anesthetics and can have minimal hypotonic or hypertonic effect on the eye.
  2. *Maintenance phase:*
     - This is done by ketamine.
     - Usually for long duration procedures such as vitreoretinal and oculoplasty surgeries
  3. *Recovery phase.*

Regional Anesthesia

Advantages:
- Simple procedure
- No pain to patient or analgesia
- No squeezing of the eyeball
- Good cooperation of the patient
- No movement of eyeball or akinesia
- Superior rectus and inferior rectus bridle sutures are possible.
- Limbal incision with cauterization is possible.
- No fear of surgery
- The cases where general anesthesia is not possible.

Disadvantages:
- Prick pain during anesthesia
- Due to akinesia, patient cannot follow the instructions of surgeon.
- Surgeon has to wait for 10–15 minutes for the effect of anesthesia.
- Patching is needed.

Complications:
- Conjunctival chemosis
- Retrobulbar hemorrhage
- Damage to optic nerve
- Globe perforation

Topical Anesthesia

Advantages:
- No prick to the patient

- Patient will obey the order by moving the eyeball to the respected direction according to the surgeons need.
- No need of postoperative patching of the eye
- Early rehabilitation of patient
- In some cases, where regional anesthesia is not indicated

Disadvantages:
- Procedure is difficult for uncooperative patients.
- Incision and capsulorhexis are sometimes difficult.
- Sometimes, movements of eyeball are uncontrolled.
- Conversion of case from phaco to small-incision cataract surgery (SICS) or extracapsular cataract extraction (ECCE) is difficult.

General Anesthesia

Advantages:
- In children
- Uncooperative patient
- In cases where there are chances of lengthy procedure

Disadvantages: All the disadvantages related to procedure and drugs of general anesthesia.

■ KEY POINTS

- According to the author, selection of anesthesia varies from case to case. Sometimes, one may need to combine these anesthesia for fruitful and good surgical outcome.
- Nowadays, topical anesthesia is the first choice for cataract surgeries.

CHAPTER 5

Bridle Sutures

■ INTRODUCTION

Bridle sutures are one of the most important steps in cataract surgery.

■ SUPERIOR RECTUS BRIDLE SUTURE

The insertion of the superior rectus is at 7.7 mm from superior limbus. One has to take the bridle suture with optimum hold of superior rectus muscle.

Instruments: Superior rectus forcep, Silcock needle holder, and 3-0 nonabsorbable black silk surgical suture with round body curved needle.

Procedure: Needle is held at the junction of the proximal one-third and distal two-thirds of it. Superior rectus forcep is designed in such a way that the angle of the holding part is kept on limbus and the tip catches the muscle perfectly.

Advantages:
- For maintaining the primary position of the globe
- Good exposure of the superior part of the globe
- All entries from the superior aspect become easy
- Incision-making steps such as the use of No. 15 blade, crescent, keratome, and conjunctival incision become easy and well approachable
- Putting viscoelastics through the incision becomes easy
- Entry of the capsulorhexis needle via the main port before starting the capsulorhexis is easy
- Entry of the phaco probe and irrigation aspiration cannula is easy
- Facilitates visco expression of soft nucleus, epinucleus, and small pieces of the nucleus

- Useful during extension of incision from 2.8 to 3 mm and from 2.8 to 6 mm for implantation of foldable and nonfoldable intraocular lenses (IOL)
- Taking suture at main incision in some circumstances is easy.
- In difficult situations, conversion of phaco to small incision cataract surgery (SICS) or extracapsular cataract surgery is possible.

INFERIOR RECTUS BRIDLE SUTURE

The inferior rectus insertion is situated at 6.5 mm from the inferior limbus.

Instruments used and the procedure for the inferior rectus is the same as for the superior rectus bridle suture.

Advantages:
- It gives counter pressure so that it hastens easy entry into anterior chamber by keratome and MVR blades.
- *Capsulorhexis*: Good red glow and primary position of the globe is must for this important step in phaco.
- Maintain the primary position of the globe, which is helpful for the following steps of nucleus management:
  - *Trench:* It can be used to maintain the primary position of the globe for better visualization, actually helps in doing this procedure due to counter pressure of inferior rectus hold and helpful to assess the last strokes of the trench.
  - Hold and chop: of each half of nucleus for better 0° effect.
  - Emulsification of small pieces—primary position helps for better phaco fluidics, which is helpful for this step.
  - Irrigation-Aspiration of epinucleus and cortex—many times we need to lift the inferior rectus for removal of the superior cortex.
- For proper placement and confirmation of an IOL in the bag.

This step is more important in following situations:
- Small palpebral fissure
- Deep socket
- Patient who continuously squeezes his or her eyes (this might be noticed during slit-lamp examination while preparing the patient).

- In unpredictable situations, where the surgeon feels that conversion of the surgery is needed.
- Combined cataract with glaucoma surgery.

■ COMPLICATIONS

- Conjunctival chemosis
- Subconjunctival hemorrhage
- Conjunctival tear
- Ptosis
- Catching oblique muscles instead of the recti with subsequent complications
- Corneal abrasion
- Postoperative pain or discomfort
- Bradycardia due to vagal stimulation is rare but a serious complication
- Scleral puncture

■ KEY POINTS

- Superior and inferior rectus bridle sutures are must for beginner phaco surgeons.
- The biggest achievement is primary position of eyeball which is important for many steps of phaco surgery.
- In difficult situations, conversion of phaco to SICS or extracapsular cataract extraction (ECCE) procedure is easy.
- According to the author, phaco surgery without these steps is like running a car without steering.

CHAPTER 6

Incision

■ INTRODUCTION
- Since it is the first step of surgery, it is important to create an ideal incision.
- Further steps of the surgery depend largely upon the incision.
- Postoperative astigmatism depends upon the incision, so after an experience of particular type of incision, it should not be changed to have surgeon's own surgically-induced astigmatism (SIA), which is important for premium lenses, especially toric lenses in practice.
- Phaco fluidics depend upon the incision. Fluidics may change with the type, position, and construction of the wound.

■ INCISIONS USED IN SURGERY
- *Main incision:*
  - Clear corneal incision
  - Limbal incision
  - Sclerocorneal incision
- *Side port incision no. I for:*
  - Chopper
  - Injection of viscoelastics
  - Bimanual irrigation aspiration
  - Rod which stabilizes eye during topical anesthesia
- *Side port incision no. II for:*
  - Capsulorhexis
  - Bimanual irrigation aspiration
  - Vitrectomy probe if required
  - Dialer and visco cannula for rotation of nucleus or intraocular lens (IOL), if needed.

■ PRINCIPLE OF INCISION (FIG. 1)
All incisions should always be directed toward the center of the eye. This is because the movement arc of the instruments is equal on both

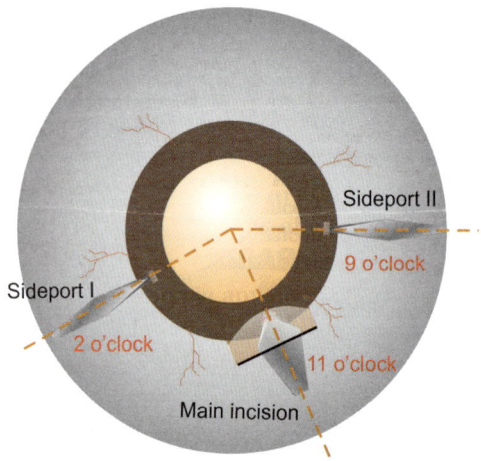

Fig. 1: Site of main and side port incision (blades are directed toward the center during the incision).

the sides from the center and thus, all the instruments can reach at any part of the eye without any hindrance offered by the ends of the incision. For this, the surgeon should be very careful while creating incision; the direction of all instruments should be exactly toward the center of the eye.

■ CONSTRUCTION OF WOUND

The incision should be valvular so that all the instruments can be smoothly inserted inside the eye and no tissue or other contents should come out easily, which is now the main factor in the surgery. Such incision gives more stability and integrity as the chamber is usually well maintained throughout surgery. An ideal wound is always necessary to prevent complications such as infection, wound leakage, shallow anterior chamber and help for IOL stability.

Architecture of Incision (Figs. 2A to E)

Following are the architecture of incision:
- Uniplanar
- Biplanar

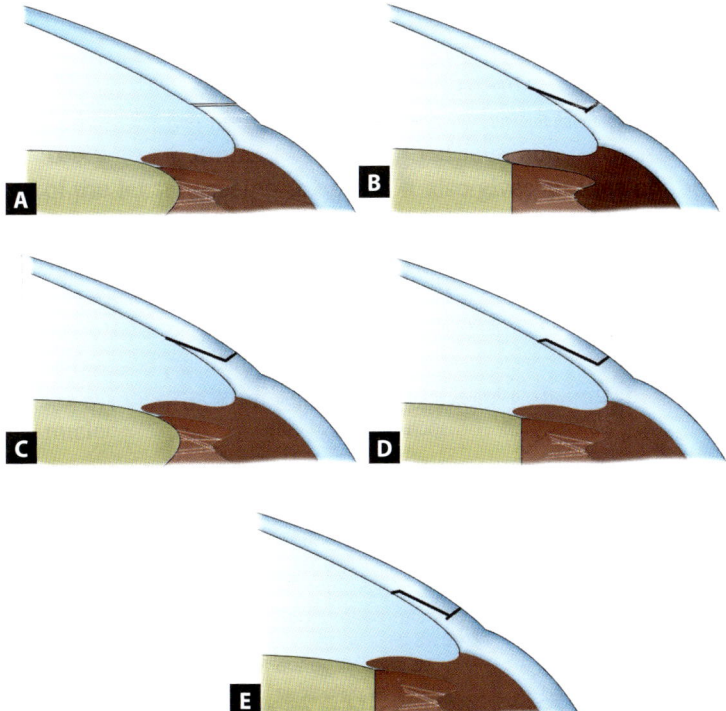

Figs. 2A to E: Architecture of incision. (A) Uniplanar; (B) Biplanar with hinge; (C) Biplanar; (D) Triplanar; and (E) Triplanar with hinge.

- Biplanar with hinge
- Triplanar
- Triplanar with hinge

Instruments used for creation of incision:
- Tooth forceps
- Conjunctival scissors
- No. 15 blade
- Crescent
- 15° blade
- *Microvitreoretinal (MVR) blade:* 19- or 20-gauge (straight or angulated)
- Keratome

■ PROCEDURE

Main Port Incision: For Limbal or Scleral (Figs. 3A to D)

- *Conjunctival cutting:*
  - *Tooth forceps:* This instrument is to hold the conjunctiva and tenons at the site of incision to be created just away from the limbus.
  - *Conjunctival scissors:* These are initially used to take a nick in the conjunctival tissue and then used to separate the conjunctiva and tenons from the sclera at 11 o'clock site.
- *Groove:*
  - *No. 15 blade:* This is used to create a partial-thickness scleral cut at the site of intended incision.
- *Tunnel:*
  - *Crescent:* This is the instrument with rounded but sharp edges used to enlarge the groove for the creation of entry through sclera and passing into layers of cornea. This instrument is useful as it directs a tunnel from the external lip to the internal lip and is the key factor for the stability of the wound.

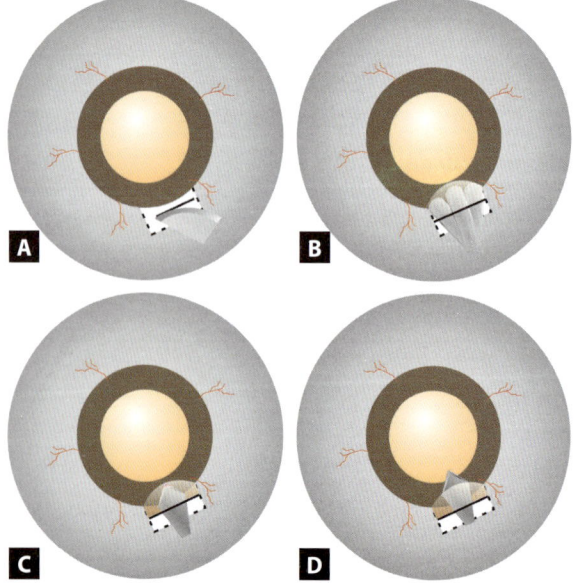

Figs. 3A to D: Limbal incision.

- **Entry in the anterior chamber:**
  - *Keratome:* This instrument with a sharp tip and edges is used to create the inner opening of the wound. It can be of various sizes, from 1.2 to 2.8 mm, which determines the size of the final inner wound that will be created. The wound size is usually decided by the surgeon and can be changed for other steps as and when required. Normally, size of the keratome is 2.00–2.8 mm.

Side port Incisions (Figs. 4A to D)

Both the side port incisions are created with the help of following instruments:

15° blade: This instrument is having pointed tip with one edge sharp and the other side blunt (sharp edge should always be directed toward surgeon).

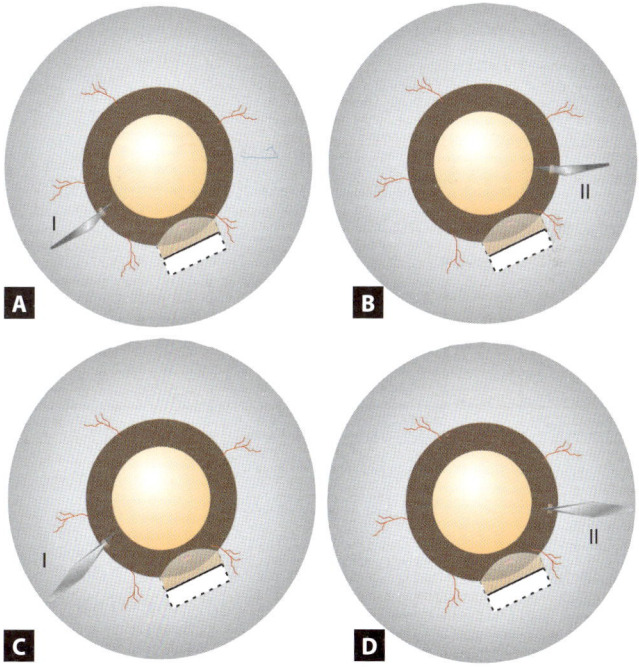

Figs. 4A to D: Side port incision.

MVR blade: This instrument has a sharp tip with cutting edges on both sides. The caliber used is 19- or 20-gauge.

Site of Incision

The main port incision is at 11 o'clock position (right-handed person), since surgeon does not have any problem in passing the phaco tip, easy manipulation, and avoiding kinking of at junction of handpiece and tubings. In other words, handling of the phaco probe is also fine and accurate, which facilitates effective procedure.

The life of the instruments, such as phaco probe, and the irrigation aspiration handpiece is also increased when they are used in this position.

Side port incision no. I is mainly used for the chopper and rod for fixation. This incision should be in the left side of the surgeon. This incision should be 90° away from the main incision so that operative manipulations of the surgeon are very comfortable by both hands. This usually happens when the surgeon uses 15° angulated blade or MVR blade and creates the side port incision at 2 o'clock position. This position also allows the synchronized and coordinated movement between phaco probe and chopper.

Side port incision no. II for the capsulorhexis is usually at 9 o'clock position. The angulation between this port and the main port should be such that these incisions should be nonparallel to each other. The nonparallel nature of this incision will prevent leak of fluid from this incision and thus prevent abnormal fluidics during the phaco surgery, which will prevent further complications such as intraoperative wound leak, forward movement of the posterior capsule, and iris prolapse. This port can also be used for bimanual irrigation aspiration and both the aspiration probe, and the irrigation probe can be used from this incision depending upon the site of cortical matter left.

The position of this incision can be changed if there is some abnormality or difficulty in creating incision at 9 o'clock position, such as pterygium, pinguecula, dense vascularization, thinning of cornea, abnormal mass in that position, anterior synechia or arcus, high nasal bridge, corneal opacity, etc.

Both side port incisions should be of adequate size and always clear corneal.

Curved MVR blade is the author's choice to prepare side port incisions.

◼ PROCEDURE

Main Port: Limbal Incision

Conjunctival flap is created by holding conjunctiva just away from the limbus with the help of toothed conjunctival grasping forceps. The aim here should be to grasp both the conjunctival and tenon in one grasp and to take a nick at conjunctiva. Following this, the scissors are passed via this nick inside the suprascleral space in closed position to separate the tissues from the sclera and open to complete this separation for a distance as required for main port incision. Following this, the separated conjunctiva and the tenon are cut from their attachment from the limbus to get sufficient space for the main port incision creation. The final shape of the conjunctival cut should be such that it remains relaxed at the edges and should also expose the required sclera for the creation of the main port incision. This conjunctival cut is usually good since it provides a good cover to the wound postoperatively, which is one of the reasons of decreased chances of infections in the limbal incision. This conjunctival cover also provides additional healing ability, stability, and strength to the incision postoperatively, thus making it a *choice of incision for the author.*

With the help of No. 15 blade, a straight-line groove is made from 10:30 to 11:30 o'clock positions at limbus. This cut should involve one third of the scleral thickness. This incision is created only with the help of superior rectus bridle suture to make a good exposure of the tissue horizontally. The angulation of the blade should be at 45°. Thus, the main aim to use this instrument is to provide a grove of sufficient depth and strength so that the surgeon can proceed with the tunnel creation with the help of crescent; thus, it should neither be too deep nor too superficial as the strength of the tunnel depends upon it.

Crescent is used to confirm the depth of the groove first. This is done by passing the sharp rounded end of the instrument under the incision made by the No. 15 blade. Following this, the crescent is moved parallel to sclera in the center of the groove with sideway movements on either side and thus, tunnel in the sclera and 1–1.5 mm into the layers of the cornea is created. Then the crescent is moved on either side of the tunnel to form adequate pockets. The total length comes out to be 3–3.5 mm. The advantage of this is that this pocket protects the side wall of the keratome and also provides the strength to the incision of the main port. The main use of crescent for the tunnel creation is that it provides the pathway for passage of the keratome and also holds the incision tight.

Keratome used in phaco practice is usually 2.00–2.8 mm in size and these are sufficient for the movement of most of the instruments passed from the main port. The keratome is passed with the cutting edge parallel to the groove created by the No. 15 blade and then extended in a tunnel made by crescent; the tip of the keratome should be at the center of the tunnel pointing toward the center of the eye, and at 1–1.5 mm from the limbus, the cornea is entered with a slight dimple at the entry site, giving a perfect triplanar shape to the incision. The keratome should then be entered to the full width of the cutting edge, taking care that the anterior chamber does not collapse and one must avoid injury to the cornea, iris, and anterior capsule by this instrument while entering. The triplanar nature of this incision makes it valvular. This is the exact specification of the limbal incision.

First Side port Incision

This is created with the help of 15° *angulated blade* or *MVR blade* usually, and it is the first entry inside the eye through which the surgeon enters the anterior chamber. To create this incision, one requires a fixed and stable eyeball which can be obtained by either tooth forceps or with the help of cotton buds or by bridle suture. These maneuvers also help in providing a perfect position of the eyeball for the creation of the incision. The principle to be kept in consideration while creating this incision is that the length of the incision by the 15° angulated blade should be greater than the width of the incision. This principle helps to create an ideal side port incision. If reverse happens, then there can be chances of complications like Descemet's membrane (DM) stripping, cornea trauma, and shallowing of anterior chamber intraoperatively. There are also chances of difficult movement of chopper via this side port incision and difficulty in chopping the pieces as required. The length of the wound should not be too large as compared to the width as it may cause more iris prolapse and leaky wound creation. This incision should also be directed toward the center of the eye.

Second Side port Incision

This is similar in most aspects to the first side port incision and is another channel to get entry into the anterior chamber. The main differences between this incision and the first side port incision are that this incision is created at the 9 o'clock position and facilitates the movement of microcapsulorhexis forceps and 26- or 30-gauge bent needle for the creation of capsulorhexis. This incision should be made with utmost care as this is the incision which governs the size and the shape of the capsulorhexis. This incision should be nonparallel to the main port incision.

Clear Corneal Incision (Fig. 5)

Diamond blades are more helpful for clear corneal incision. Keratome, side port blade, used for this step should be sharp.

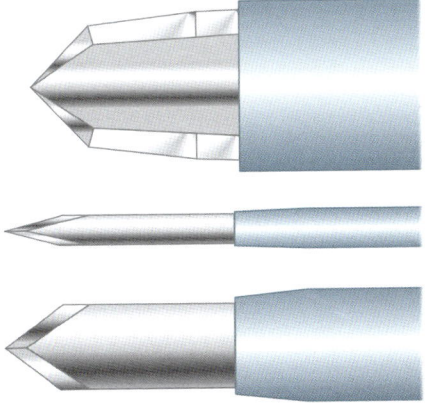

Fig. 5: Diamond blades.

Clear Corneal Main Port Incision (Figs. 6A to C)

- This incision is also a triplanar or biplanar incision but is less valvular as compared to the limbal incision. This can be created by keratome only or with the help of crescent and keratome depending upon the surgeons. Procedure is same as mentioned earlier for main port for limbal incision. These incisions are leaky and usually require a stitch.
- **Figures 7A to F** show clear corneal main incision.

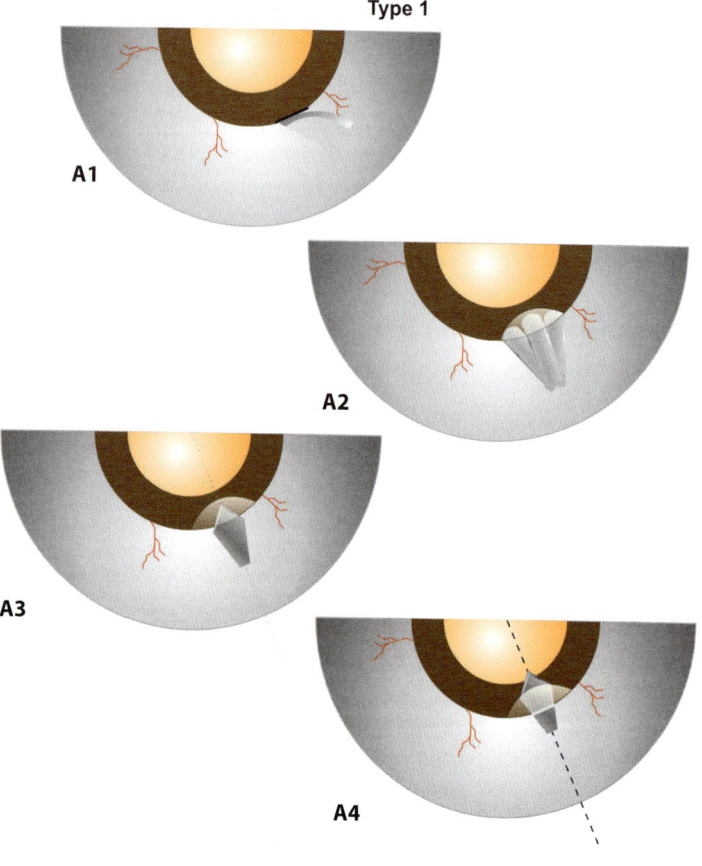

Fig. 6A

Type 2

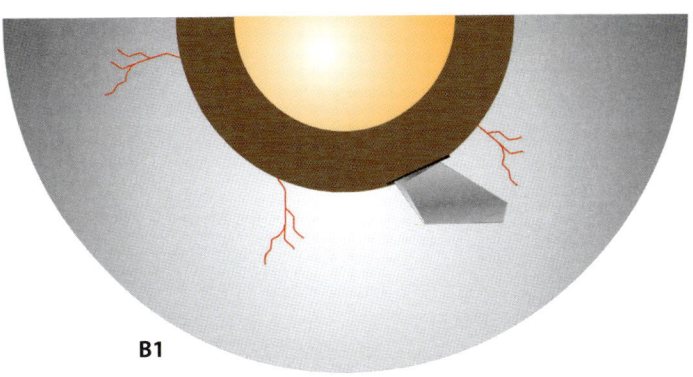

B1

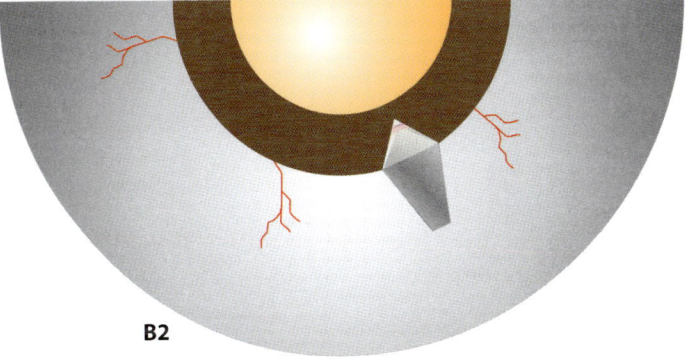

B2

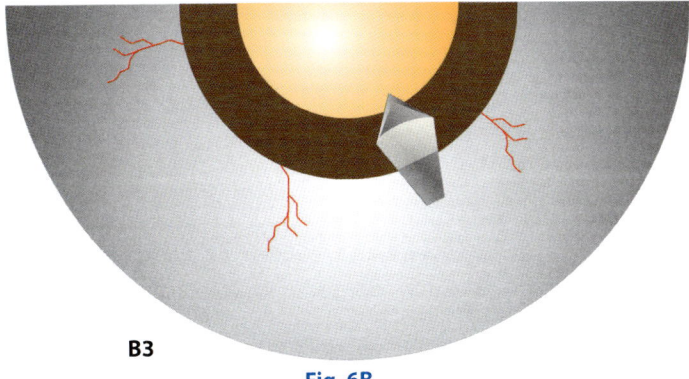

B3

Fig. 6B

Incision

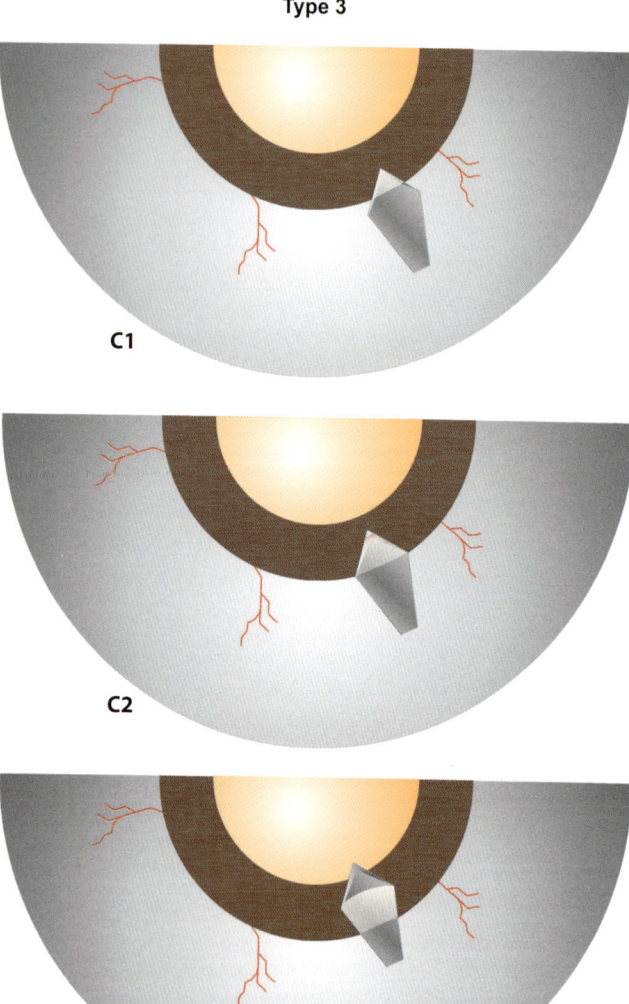

Figs. 6A to C: (A1) 15 No. blade; (A2) Crescent; and (A3 and A4) Keratome; (B) Clear corneal incision: (B1 and B2) Start the groove with keratome and (B3) incision completed by keratome; (C) Clear corneal incision: (C1 and C2) Direct entry by keratome and (C3) incision completed by keratome.

ADVANTAGES AND DISADVANTAGES OF DIFFERENT TYPES OF MAIN PORT INCISION

Limbal-type Main Port Incision

Advantages

- Incision is covered by the conjunctiva
- Lesser chances of postoperative infection
- A perfect triplanar incision with good valvular effect
- Stronger wound architecture
- Near to required square configuration of incision
- Conversion to small-incision cataract surgery (SICS) is easier with these incisions
- Stability of the anterior chamber is more
- Phaco fluidics is better
- Conversion from foldable lens to nonfoldable lens is easy and natural with this type of incision
- It is astigmatically neutral incision
- Healing is faster as compared to the clear corneal incision.

Disadvantages

- Peribulbar anesthesia is required, and it may or may not be done under topical anesthesia.
- Pain is more with this type of incision.
- Conjunctiva is cut and there may be red eye for few days.
- Chemosis is usually present.
- Cosmetically more depressing.
- More instrumentation is required.
- Difficult as more skill is required.

Conditions where limbal incision is not advised:

- Scleritis or sclerosing keratitis
- Post retinal detachment-treated cases
- Post glaucoma surgery cases
- Post pterygium surgery where conjunctival flap is taken for autograft.

Clear Corneal Incision

Advantages

- Surgery under topical anesthesia is possible

- Easy to perform
- Lesser instrumentation
- Faster speed of surgery
- More comfortable
- More movement of instruments is possible
- Ideal for deep socket and narrow palpebral fissure
- Phaco tip is near to nucleus, so workup is easy.

Disadvantages

- Less valvular so less stable
- Astigmatism may be more if architecture is not perfect
- Leaky and takes more time to heal
- Fluidics may be poorer
- Stitches may be required
- More chances of infection due to directly exposed wound.

CORRELATION OF PHACO FLUIDICS WITH INCISION

Flow rate is one of the most important factors and is governed by the architecture of both main port and side port incisions. It should always be kept in mind that wrong incision and leaky wounds, can hamper flow rate and then surgery can be difficult. Instrumentation inside the eye is difficult; posterior capsule always keeps coming near to the instruments, so the chances of posterior capsular rent are more, followability of the tissue is less as compared to that in a closed wound, more burns are seen in the cornea in such cases, and the chances of trauma to the cornea are more.

CORRELATION OF INCISION WITH IRIS MOVEMENT

Wound or incision of bad architecture is usually associated with more chances of iris prolapse which may need a suture at the site to prevent postoperative complications. Once the memory of iris is lost, it is difficult to reposition it without risk of future iris prolapsed and further damage. This should be remembered while deciding about whether to take suture in such cases at the end of surgery. One must always aim at creating an incision which is so sound that it should avoid any movement, trauma, and manipulation of the iris.

KEY POINTS

- Incision is the first step to start phaco, so it should be perfect technically to make it valvular.
- Phaco fluidics depends on architecture of incision.
- Use of sharp blades for incision is mandatory.

LIVE SURGERY PHOTOGRAPHS

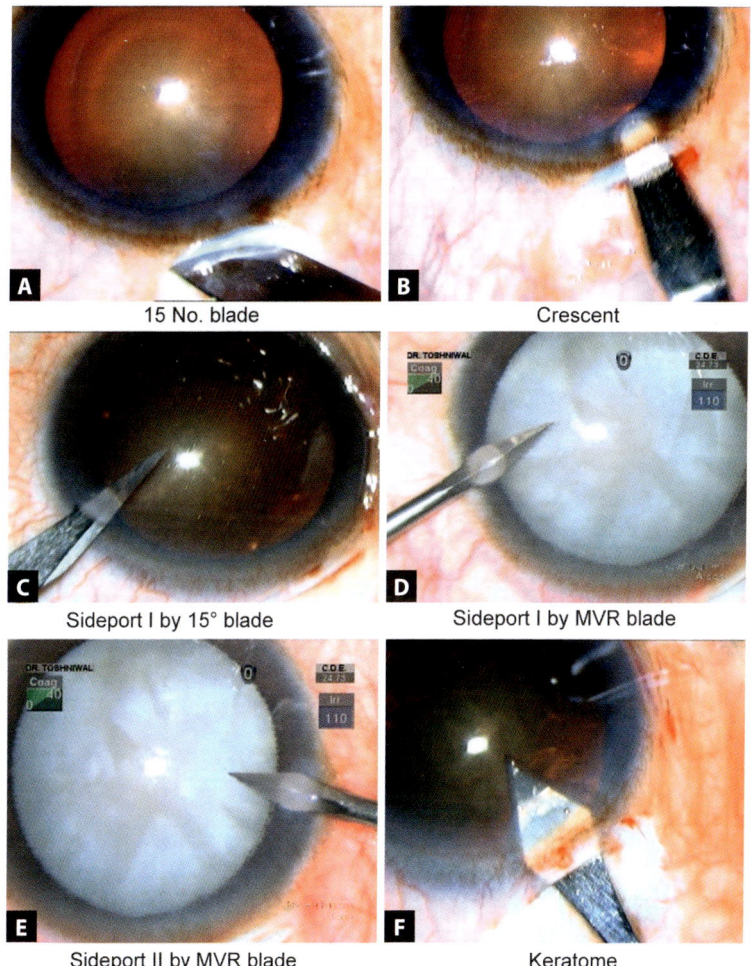

Figs. 7A to F: Incision. (MVR: microvitreoretinal)

CHAPTER 7

Capsulorhexis

■ INTRODUCTION

Capsulorhexis is the process of peeling of the anterior capsule of the lens in a central continuous curvilinear fashion.

It is one of the most important steps in phacoemulsification. Surgeons cannot start surgery in a confident and predictable way unless capsulorhexis is completed.

According to the author, it is not only important to do capsulorhexis but also to start to feel it.

■ ANATOMICAL CONSIDERATION (FIG. 1)

The total diameter of the human lens is 9–10 mm. The insertion of the zonules occurs at 2 mm on anterior side and 1 mm on the posterior side; thus, there is an area of 7 mm. Sometimes, plus or

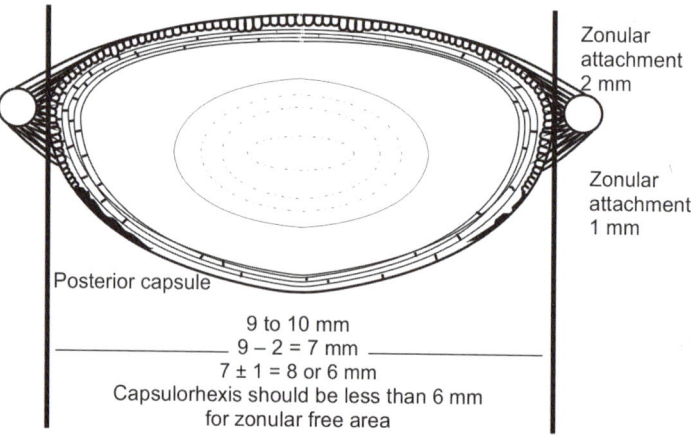

Fig. 1: Anatomy of the lens with capsule. Anterior capsule with basement membrane with epithelial cells.

minus 1 mm means 6 mm, which is actually a zonule-free area. For safety and the size of the optic of an intraocular lens (IOL), ideally the capsulorhexis should be about 4.5–5.5 mm in diameter, with 0.5 mm on either side for practical purposes.

The author prefers an adequate-sized capsulorhexis (4.5–5.5 mm).

Variations in the size of the capsulorhexis may be related to variations in the anatomy of the lens and the eye.

■ PREREQUISITES (FIG. 2)

- *Flat anterior capsule:* This is one of the most important prerequisites for capsulorhexis because it provides the surgeon with a better control during this important step.
- A convex anterior capsule, on the other hand, will make it too difficult for a surgeon to do capsulorhexis.
- High anterior chamber (AC) pressure in comparison to an intrabag pressure
- Normal AC depth
- Primary position of the eyeball

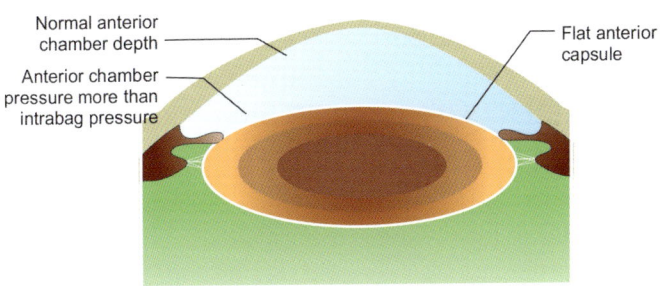

Fig. 2: Prerequisite for capsulorhexis.

■ PHYSICS OF CAPSULORHEXIS (FIGS. 3A AND B)

Tear by Stretching

- The force is in the plane of maximum resistance.
- Force is directed perpendicular to the desired direction of tearing.
- Tear in this way moves rapidly and uncontrolled.

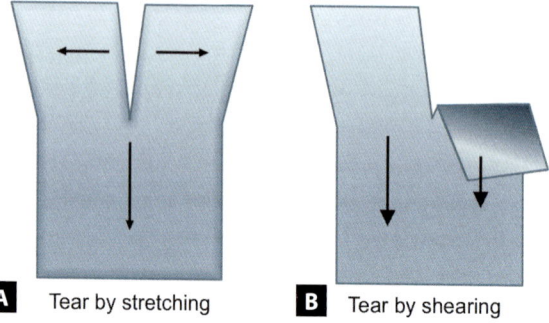

Figs. 3A and B: Physics of capsulorhexis.

Results:
- Capsulorhexis is not under control of surgeons
- Chances of running away of capsule toward equator are common.

Tear by Shearing
- The force is in the plane of least resistance
- Force is directed parallel to the desired direction of tearing
- Tear in this way moves slowly and is controlled.

Result: Capsulorhexis is under better control of surgeon.

■ INSTRUMENTS (FIGS. 4A TO E)
- *Cystitome:* A 26- or 30-gauge bent needle or insulin syringe with needle
- Capsulorhexis forceps used via the main port
- Microcapsulorhexis forceps used via side port
- Microscissors
- Vannas scissors

Cystitomes
- These are usually 26- or 30-gauge needles which are sharp and thin and are constructed in a way to perform capsulorhexis.
- Cystitomes are useful for giving the initial nick in the anterior capsule.

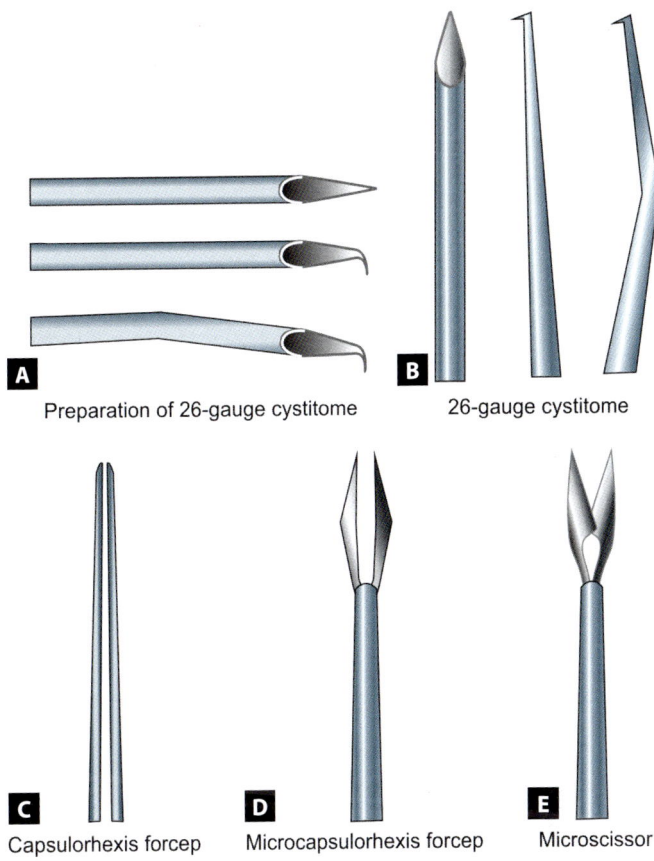

Figs. 4A to E: Instruments.

- The aim here is to give a shape to the needle so that the tip can do the work of capsulorhexis and the shaft of the needle helps to fit in contour of the cornea, with the help of the needle holder.
- First bend is at the junction of distal one third and proximal two thirds of the bevel part of the tip, at approximately 90° with the bevel side facing up. This bend tip length is dependent on the AC depth and also on the capsule architecture.
- The second bend is given at the base of the needle which is also at 90° to the shaft of the needle.

- The third bend is in the middle part of the needle which is performed to give the final contour simulating that of the cornea.
  - Normally, this needle is mounted upon a 2-cc syringe.
  - Cystitomes can be used with a syringe-filled viscoelastics or saline, which can also be used to maintain the AC depth with AC maintainer.

Advantages

- Simple instrument
- Easy to prepare
- Cheap
- First nick is easy to do
- AC is well-maintained
- Visibility is not hampered during the procedure.
- Closed chamber technique of the capsulorhexis
- Being a closed chamber technique, control on the anterior capsule is better in the first part of the capsulorhexis.
- Cystitome can be passed through a small opening.
- In a preexisting shallow AC, cystitome is more helpful.

Disadvantages

- More chances of Descemet's detachment at the incision site
- Chances of endothelial touch with the needle
- Chances of injury to the iris is also common, which may lead to small pupil.
- If the AC collapses during the procedure, the needle can puncture or tear the anterior capsule at a different site, which leads to difficulty in completing the capsulorhexis.
- During the last part of the capsulorhexis, if capsule runs away to the periphery, then chances of control are less.
- Control on the anterior capsule is less as compared to the forceps, as you can grasp both surfaces of the capsule using the forceps, which is not possible with using the cystitome.
- The procedure may be difficult when the pupil gets small during the procedure.
- In mature cataracts, there is less control on the capsule after the first nick.

Forceps Used Via Main Port
- Utrata forceps or other capsulorhexis forceps
- These instruments are introduced via the main port.

Advantages
- The capsulorhexis performed with this instrument is more controlled as compared to 26-gauge needle.
- Completing capsulorhexis which has been started with a cystitome
- In some situations, like mature cataract, hard cataracts, and subluxated cataracts, where one needs more control on the capsule
- If capsulorhexis runs away, it can be easily managed with the Vannas scissors and the capsulorhexis forceps through the main port.
- Reconsideration of the size and shape of the capsule is very well-managed in the last part of the capsulorhexis.

Disadvantages
- Requires a main port which is about 2.8 mm section
- Shallowing of the AC while using this instrument
- In a deep socket and in a narrow palpebral fissure, passing this instrument through the main port is very difficult.

Forceps via Side Port
Microcapsulorhexis forceps: This forceps works in a dual way.

This instrument can be passed like a needle through a small opening and works as a forceps and thus has the advantage of both needle and forceps. The author has invented a unique design called Toshniwal microcapsulorhexis forceps which is his instrument of choice for this step.

Advantages
All advantages which have been mentioned earlier related to forceps passed through the main port and the follows:
- Very easy instrumentation
- AC is maintained while doing this procedure.

- Helpful in difficult situations
- Prevents running away of the capsulorhexis

Disadvantage
- Expensive instrument

■ SOLUTIONS

Trypan Blue
- It is useful in staining the anterior capsule.
- *Advantages:*
  - Better visualization of the capsule, especially in mature cataract, hard cataract, and pseudoexfoliation
  - Useful in the early practice of capsulorhexis
- *Situations in which we should avoid the use of trypan blue:*
  - Hazy cornea
  - If the surgeon is planning to implant a hydrophilic acrylic IOL which may stain

Method of Staining
- Create the side port incision I or may be side port II at the same time if anterior depth is normal.
- Inject trypan blue using the undiluted solution in 2 cc syringe with a small canula.
- Now, inject air bubble via 2 cc syringe and canula fixed on it.
- Following this, again inject trypan blue which will stay under the air support.
- Time duration for keeping the dye to stain the anterior capsule varies from surgeon to surgeon but should be as minimum as possible.
- Normally, the proposed time is 10–15 seconds.
- Following this, the viscoelastics are used to fill the AC and maintain the AC depth after removal of dye via the side port.
- Create side port incision II at this point if not created before.
- Excess dye can also be removed via second side port or the main port as per the surgeon's choice.
- Air bubble which has entered during above manipulation should be removed by viscoelastics before the start of procedure.

Capsulorhexis

■ TECHNIQUE OF CAPSULORHEXIS (FIGS. 5A TO D)

- The cystitome is introduced via the side port after filling the AC with viscoelastics.
- Make a nick in the center of the anterior capsule and elevate the flap.

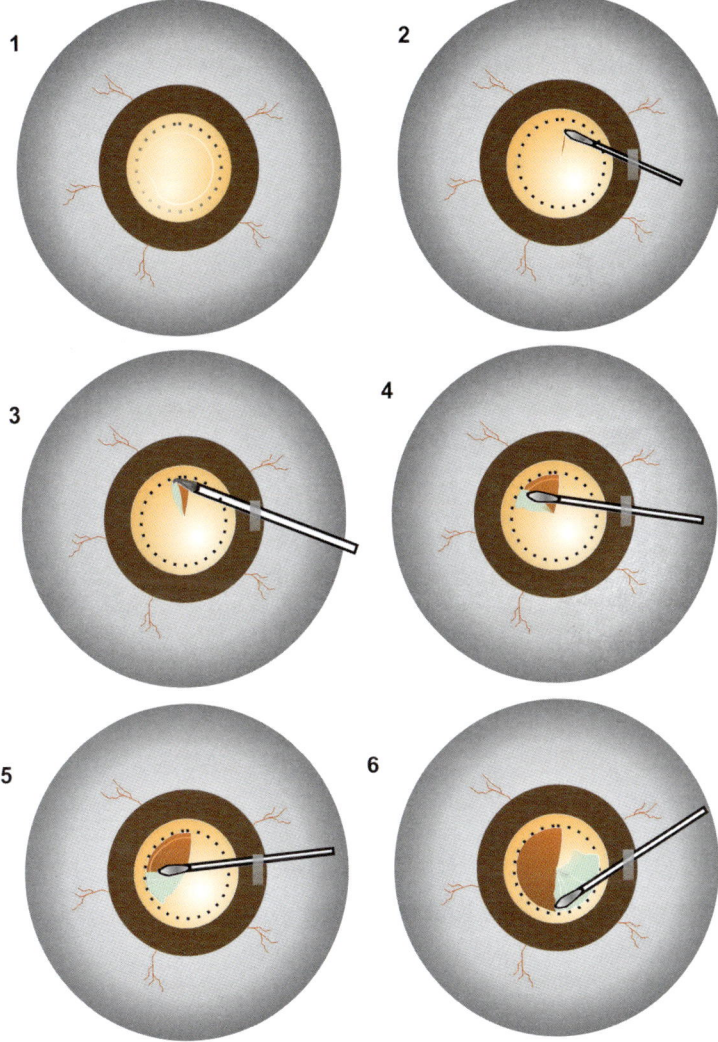

Fig. 5A

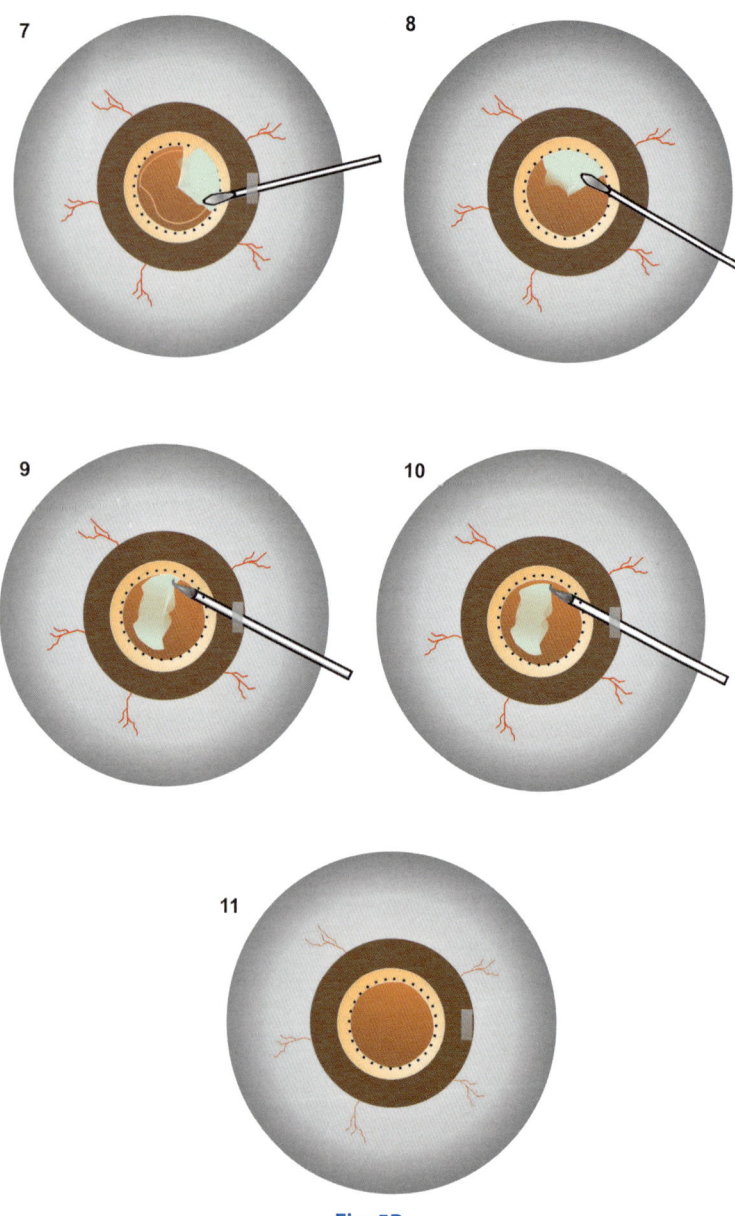

Fig. 5B

Capsulorhexis

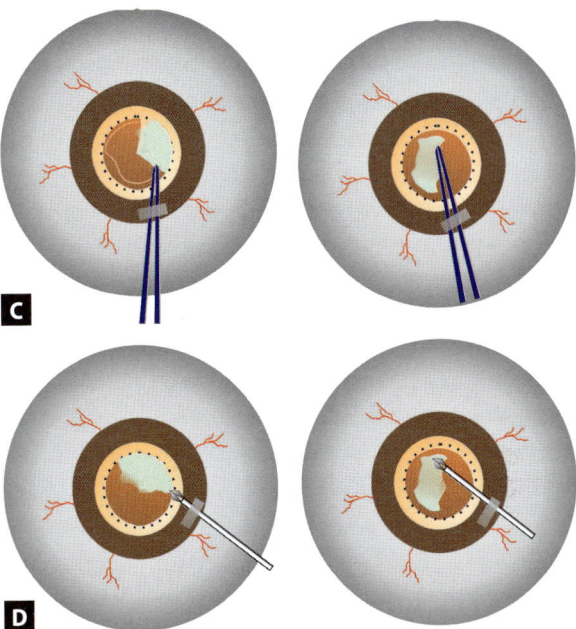

Figs. 5C and D

Figs. 5A to D: Technique of capsulorhexis: (A and B) Capsulorhexis by 26-gauge cystitome; (C) Capsulorhexis is completed by capsulorhexis forceps; and (D) Capsulorhexis is completed by microcapsulorhexis forceps.

- The direction of the flap is toward 6 o'clock when done through the right-side port and 9 o'clock when done through the left-side port (if side port is at 10 o'clock, then the direction of the nick in capsulorhexis is toward 7 o'clock), and is continued in an anticlockwise direction.
- In the author's opinion, during capsulorhexis, five important points should be taken into consideration.
    1. Better visualization of the procedure
    2. Complete watching on the torn capsule
    3. AC depth should be maintained throughout the procedure.
    4. Direction of the capsulorhexis should always be parallel to pupil.
    5. Keep the capsule relaxed, which can be achieved by putting the viscoelastics in a specific way and direction.

ZONES OF THE CAPSULORHEXIS (FIG. 6)

Zone I (6 o'clock to 3 o'clock)

This zone is the most important zone as it is the start of the capsulorhexis, where the author feels that every surgeon should take the opportunity to feel the capsule.
- Go to the base of the torned capsule with the tip of the cystitome.
- It is easy to perform the capsulorhexis here because the AC is full and the cystitome is straight and the flap is small and so the movement is controlled. Also, this area is away from incision, so there is a long arc of movement for the instrument.
- Movement should be parallel to pupil.
- AC depth should be maintained.

Zone II (3 o'clock to 12 o'clock)
- Many surgeons are scared of extension of the capsulorhexis in this zone, so they unnecessarily make it too small, so one should try to keep the adequate size of the capsulorhexis in the superior zone.

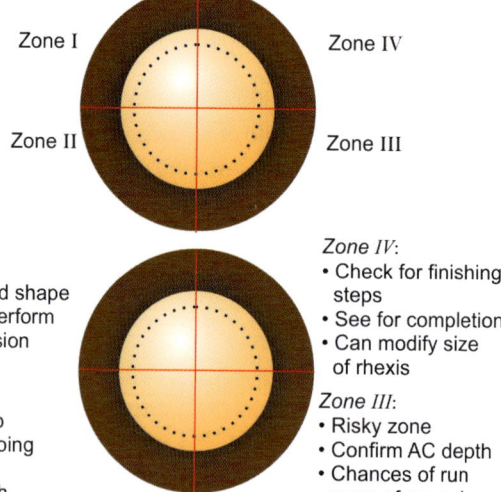

Zone I:
- Feel the rhexis
- See for size and shape
- Easy zone to perform
- Away from incision

Zone II:
- Scared to do so surgeons are doing small rhexis
- Check AC depth

Zone IV:
- Check for finishing steps
- See for completion
- Can modify size of rhexis

Zone III:
- Risky zone
- Confirm AC depth
- Chances of run away of capsule

Fig. 6: Points to remember during capsulorhexis in different zones. (AC: anterior chamber)

- Check the AC depth, if it is maintained, continue with zone III, otherwise come out with precautions not to extend the capsulorhexis in the periphery.

Zone III (12 o'clock to 9 o'clock)
- This is the risky zone.
- Confirm the AC depth before performing capsulorhexis in this zone.
- This zone is difficult for capsulorhexis procedure because:
  - The flap is near to the main incision.
  - The AC depth is difficult to maintain.
  - The capsulorhexis and the flap run away fast.
  - The flap gets larger in size.

Zone IV (9 o'clock to 6 o'clock)
- This is the finishing zone for capsulorhexis.
- Surgeon is always confident and happy at this point, but according to the author one should not be overconfident and casual.
- One can modify the size of the capsulorhexis in this zone.
- See for completion.

■ SPEED OF THE CAPSULORHEXIS (FIG. 7)
- Start the capsulorhexis with an adequate speed at the center, because if the capsulorhexis speed is high, there are more chances of run away, and if it is too slow, there may be a chance of disturbing the subcapsular cortex, which will in turn disturb the visualization and difficulty may start.
- After the first nick, in zone I, the speed is always adequate and then stops for a while to assess the AC depth and the size and shape of the capsulorhexis.
- In zone II, the speed should be relatively slower to give good contour to the capsulorhexis in the sense of adequate size and shape.
- In zone III, the speed of the capsulorhexis is relatively higher as chances of running away of the capsule are quite common as the capsulorhexis margin is near to the main site incision.
- In zone IV, the speed of the capsulorhexis should be adequate or relatively slow for better completion of the capsulorhexis with respect to the final size and shape.

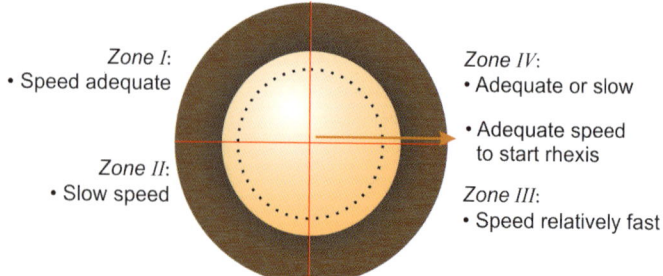

Fig. 7: Speed of the capsulorhexis.

According to the author for a successful practice of capsulorhexis, one has to have complete knowledge regarding the technique and the speed of the capsulorhexis in different zones, and the ability to use both the cystitome and the capsulorhexis forcep whenever needed.

■ VISCOELASTICS IN CAPSULORHEXIS

The use of these solutions is a must in capsulorhexis because they maintain the AC depth, which is one of the important prerequisites for this procedure.

Putting the viscoelastics through different ports of the incision is an art in the sense that every time the surgeon should keep the anatomy of the flap back to its anatomical position, or keep the flap in a relaxed position.

Sometimes during removal of the cystitome, the AC gets collapsed and this instrument being sharp can tear the anterior capsule at different sites, so to avoid this, viscoelastics can be put through another side port to maintain the AC depth.

Different Types of Viscoelastics

Cohesive

- They have high molecular weight.
- More capacity to maintain space in the eye
- Can be easily aspirated after completion of surgery
- *Commercially available solution:* Healon, Healon GV, Amvisc and Amvisc plus, hyaluron, Aurogel, Viscoat (mixture of chondroitin sulfate and sodium hyaluronate)

Dispersive
- Less tendency to escape from AC
- Difficult to remove completely from AC at the end of surgery
- *Commercially available solution:* Hydroxypropyl methylcellulose (HPMC)

Hydroxypropyl Methylcellulose
As it is a low-viscosity solution, maintaining the AC depth is always challenging for the surgeon, so to overcome this problem, one can do:
- Frequent refilling of the AC
- Putting the visco through the side port incision
- Cystitome is the preferred instrument for capsulorhexis than the capsulorhexis forceps
- Resistance to the movement of the cystitome is less.
- It is a cheap solution.
- Air bubbles and other debris can be easily removed during the procedure by the HPMC.
- It is easy to move the instruments for capsulorhexis as the viscosity is less.
- Better to do the capsulorhexis with the cystitome as the AC has to be maintained again and again.

Sodium Hyaluronate
- It is a high-molecular-weight and high-viscosity solution.
- It is a high-viscosity solution, so the AC depth is maintained for a longer duration, so this solution is the solution of choice for capsulorhexis.
- Both cystitome and forceps can be used for the capsulorhexis with this solution.
- *Anatomical* situations such as mature cataract, hard cataract, pseudoexfoliation, subluxated cataracts—this solution is the preferred solution than HPMC.
- The biggest advantage of this high-viscosity solution is in pediatric and young cataract patients, where the elasticity of the capsule is more.

- Because the viscosity of this solution is more, restricted movements of the instrument are noted during the procedure sometimes.
- Control on the capsule is better.

Combination of chondroitin sulfate and sodium hyaluronate is the choice of solution for capsulorhexis, although it is costly.

■ ANATOMICAL VARIATIONS

Hazy Cornea

- Avoid trypan blue as it may stain the cornea.
- Be careful while passing the instruments as chances of injury to the cornea, iris, and the capsule are more.

Shallow Anterior Chamber

- Putting the viscoelastic is just to maintain the AC. Sometimes, we may put more viscoelastics than the volume of the AC which may cause iris to prolapse and chances of running away of capsulorhexis is more as it becomes tense.
- Capsulorhexis should be done through the side port incision only.
- Capsulorhexis should be small, as the shallow AC is usually associated with a convex anterior capsule and many times, it is also associated with a small pupil.

Pseudoexfoliation

- Capsulorhexis should be done inside the pseudoexfoliation ring.
- Small capsulorhexis is needed as many cases are associated with small pupil and zonular weakness.

Mature Cataract

- Trypan blue is important for better visualization of the capsule.
- Forceps are preferred than the cystitome in these situations.
- High-viscosity solutions are better than HPMC.
- Try to start with small capsulorhexis so that completion of the capsulorhexis is easy.

Hypermature Cataract

First, do small capsulorhexis with microcapsulorhexis forceps. Then liquified cortex is aspirated via 5 cc syringe with cannula for decompression. Now, refill AC with viscoelastic and cut the capsule with Toshniwal microscissor and complete the capsulorhexis.

Convex Anterior Capsule

- Small capsulorhexis should be done.
- Capsulorhexis can run away at any point.

■ HOW TO PRACTICE CAPSULORHEXIS

- Used IOL box with cover of plastic can be used to do practice of capsulorhexis with cystitome.
- Training of this step is by Kitaro kit which is developed by Dr Junsuke Akura from Japan.

■ RUNNING AWAY OF THE CAPSULORHEXIS (FIG. 8)

- If run away is at more than one place or point one should usually avoid phaco surgery and may consider conversion to a small-incision cataract surgery (SICS) or extracapsular cataract extraction (ECCE), according to the situation.
- If run away is present and the nucleus is hard and big, then one must convert the case.
- If extension of the capsulorhexis or running away is at the distal 180° apart from the incision, one should avoid phaco.
- Capsulorhexis running away at proximal 180° from incision, one can consider phaco with modification.

■ KEY POINTS

- Continuous curvilinear capsulorhexis is must before start of phaco surgery.
- If capsulorhexis runs away, one can think of conversion of phaco to SICS or ECCE or do phaco surgery with precaution.
- The author insists that every surgeon should start to take feel of capsulorhexis.

Capsulorhexis

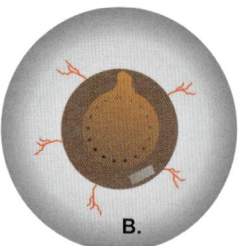
Direct pressure during trench

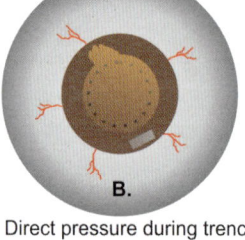
Direct pressure during trench

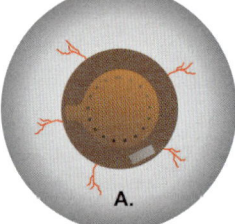
Trench on right side (Paracentral)
Right hemispher of nucleus
should be managed first

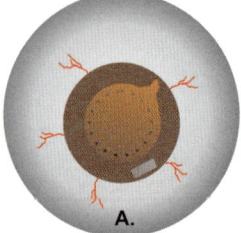
Trench on left side (Paracentral)
Left hemispher of nucleus
should be managed first

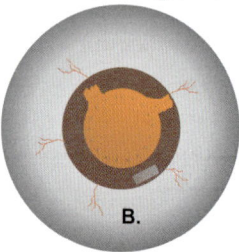
Rhexis runs away at more
than one point

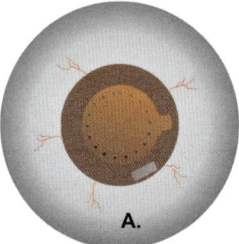
Trench on left side (Paracentral)
Left hemisphere of nucleus should be managed first

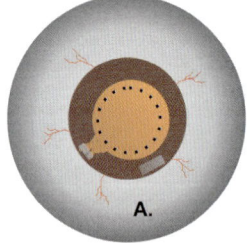
Avoid excessive manipulation
at side port incision

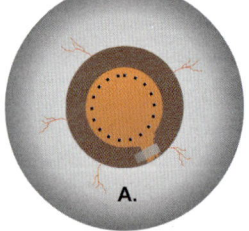
Avoid excessive manipulation
at main incision site

Fig. 8: Capsulorhexis run away: A—can do phaco;
B—unpredictable to do phaco.

Capsulorhexis

■ LIVE SURGERY PHOTOGRAPHS (FIGS. 9A TO P)

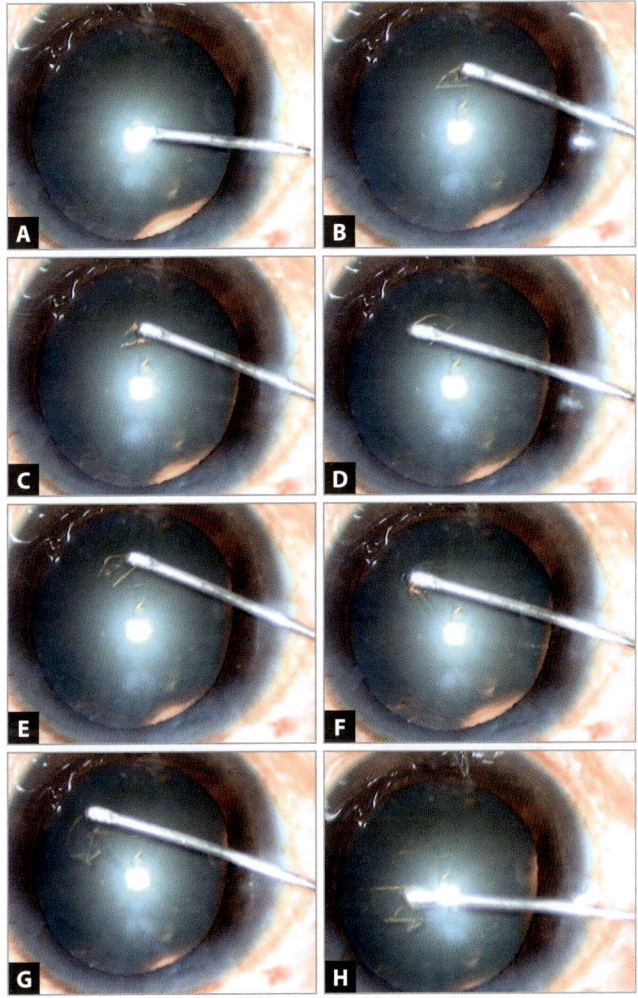

Figs. 9A to H: (A) Rhexis starting from center through side port. Puncture of the anterior capsule with cystitome; (B) Creation of capsular flap with lifting of the capsule; (C) After lifting, go at the base of the flap for further steps; (D) Direction of the flap should be parallel to the pupillary border (keeping in mind, draw a circle within a circle); (E) Again back to the base of the flap; (F) Adequate movement of the cystitome to prepare the rhexis at this place; (G) Continue the rhexis with direction of flap and needle parallel to pupillary border; (H) Shearing forces are working, so it is a well-controlled rhexis.

Capsulorhexis

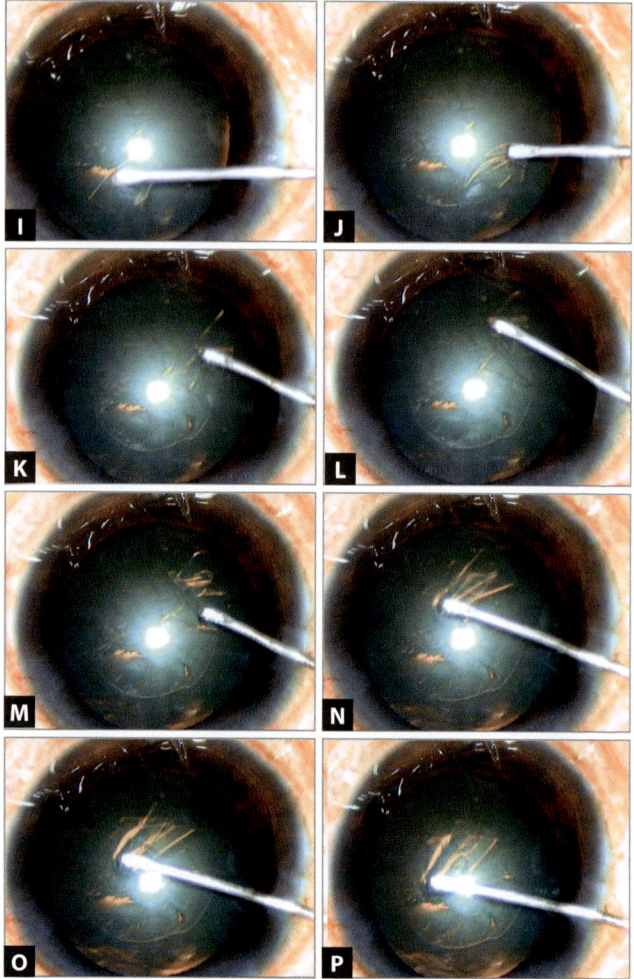

Figs. 9I to P: (I) Half rhexis is completed, check for anterior chamber; (J) Tearing of the capsule away from the base—this helps in increasing the size of rhexis; (K) Speed of the rhexis and movement of cystitome are slightly fast as rhexis is near the incision; (L) AC depth is maintained due to which rhexis is under control. Rhexis is near completion, so the cystitome which is away from the base should be now placed back to the base of flap; (M) Cystitome is now at base of the flap for completion of the rhexis in a controlled manner; (N) Tearing of the capsule with adequately deep AC depth; (O) In finishing steps, visualization of the tear should be always clear; (P) Rhexis completed of adequate size and shape.

Hydroprocedures

■ INTRODUCTION

Hydroprocedures are used for separation of layers of lens by fluid.

This is important step for rotation of lens and to avoid pressure on zonules.

■ DEFINITION (FIG. 1)

- *Hydrodelineation:* Separation between inner hard core of nucleus and adjacent epinucleus
- *Hydrodelamination:* Separation of the lens at different zones of epinucleus
- *Hydrodissection:* Separation of the cortex and capsule.

■ PROCEDURE (FIGS. 2 AND 3)

Hydrodelineation

- A 2 cc syringe filled with balanced salt solution (BSS) with beveled cannula is used for hydrodelineation.

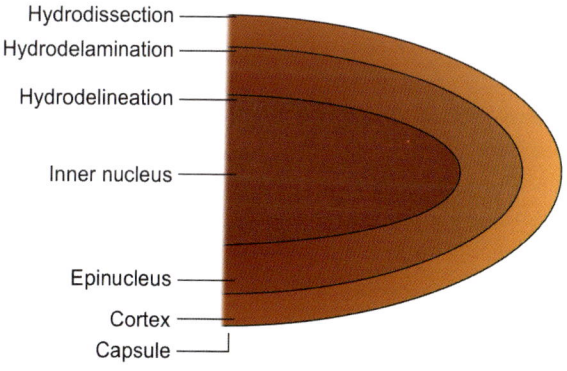

Fig. 1: Hydroprocedures.

Hydroprocedures

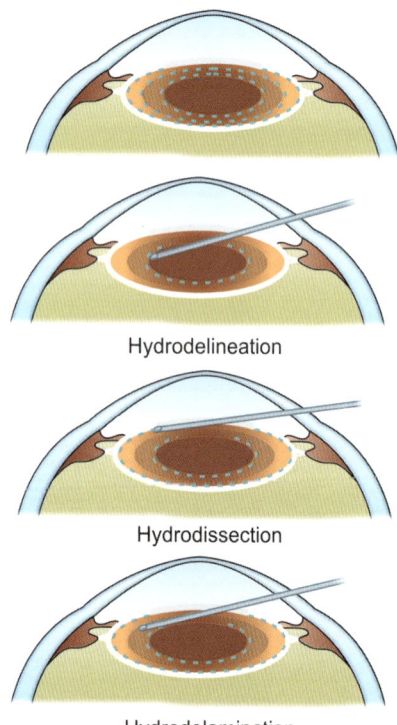

Fig. 2: Procedure: Site of hydrodelineation, hydrodissection, and hydrodelamination.

- Fill the anterior chamber with viscoelastics to normal depth so that the anatomy of the lens will be at its position, which is very important to reach specific points of separation of layers.
- In shallow anterior chamber, one cannot reach proper anatomical plain, and anterior chamber can still become shallower and this restricts the further hydroprocedures.
- Needle should pass first toward the left side of the nucleus which is more approachable for incision at 11 o'clock position.
- Pass the needle behind the capsulorhexis and in the substance of lens to reach at border of hard core of nucleus and pass the fluid very slowly and as the separation starts, one can tap the nucleus and pass more fluid to complete hydrodelineation.
- Final result is visualization of the golden ring.

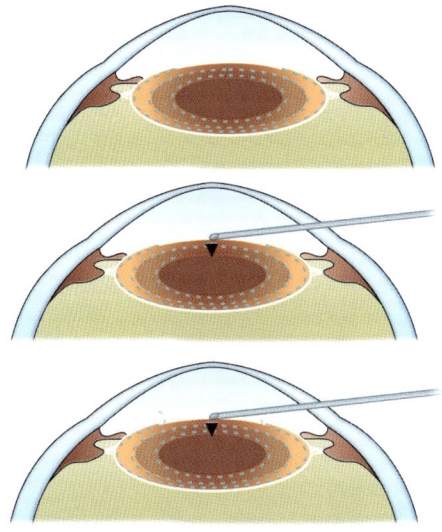

Fig. 3: Procedure (tapping of the nucleus posteriorly).

Hydrodelamination

During hydrodelineation, water current sometimes passes through the layers of epinucleus, so along with typical golden ring, one can see one to two more rings of separation of various layers of epinucleus. This is hydrodelamination.

Hydrodissection

- Pass the needle behind the anterior capsule and push the fluid parallel to the anterior capsule.
- This will separate the capsular bag from the cortex.
- This water current will move from one plain to the other and classical fluid wave can be seen. This is the sign of completion of hydrodissection.
- Following this, the nucleus is tapped at the center toward the posterior capsule to avoid capsulolenticular block.

■ COMPLICATION (FIG. 4)

Capsulolenticular block is the most dreaded complication in which complete bag with lens can fall into the vitreous cavity.

Hydroprocedures

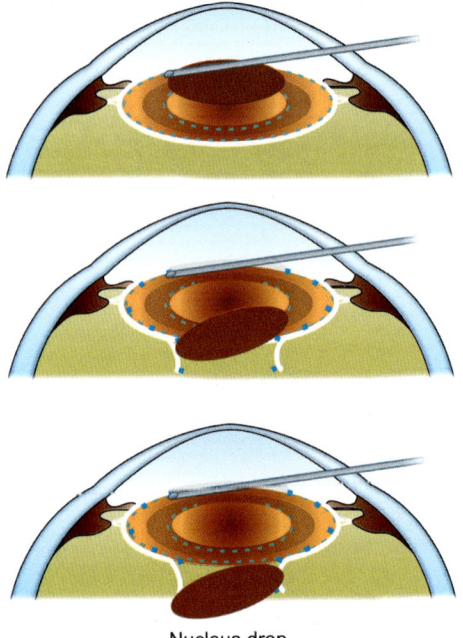

Fig. 4: Capsulolenticular block (nucleus drop).

◼ ADVANTAGES
- Rotation of nucleus is easy
- Less stress on zonules during lens management

◼ DISADVANTAGES
- Unnecessary intrabag manipulation
- Trench on mobile nucleus is difficult
- Hydroprocedures sometimes increase the intrabag pressure
- Due to soft tissue disturbance, visualization during surgery is difficult.

◼ KEY POINTS
- Golden ring is a sign of hydrodelineation.
- Classical fluid wave is a sign of hydrodissection.
- Adequate hydroprocedure is ideal.
- Excessive hydroprocedure is not recommended by the author.

Hydroprocedures

■ LIVE SURGERY PHOTOGRAPHS (FIGS. 5A TO F)

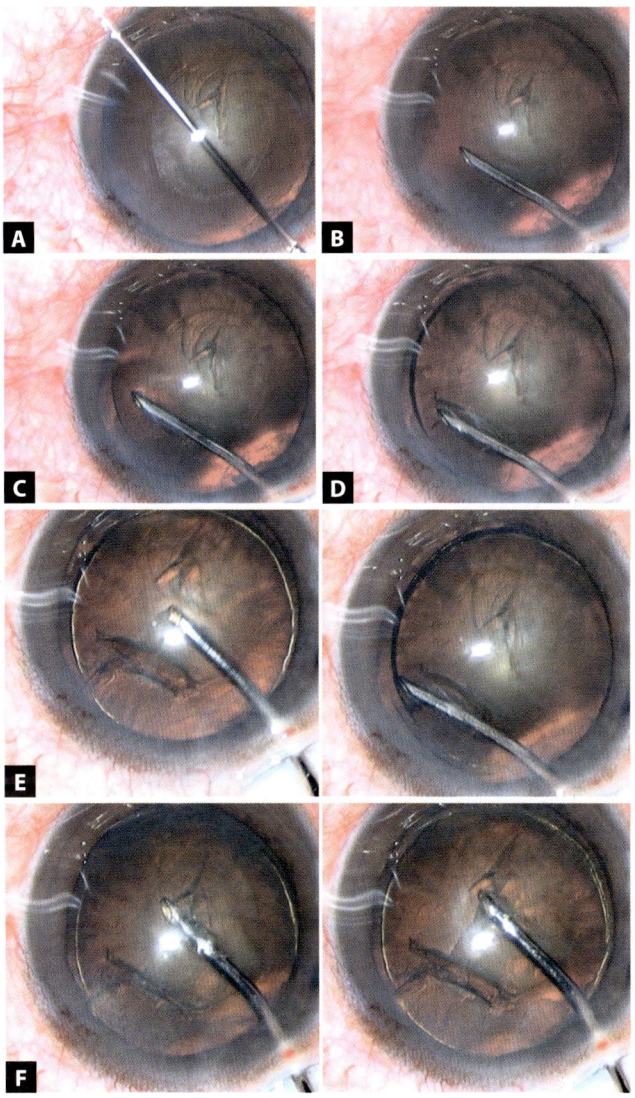

Figs. 5A to F: (A) Confirm the direction and speed of water flow outside; (B) Placement of the hydrocannula beneath the capsulorhexis in the deeper layers of the nucleus; (C) Water is injected slowly; (D) Cleavage starts between nucleus and epinucleus; (E) Formation of the golden ring is a sign of complete hydrodelineation; and (F) Decompression of the bag by tapping the central part of nucleus to avoid capsule lenticular block.

CHAPTER 9

Trench

■ INTRODUCTION

Trench is sculpting of nucleus. This is the first step where surgeon actually, feels the nucleus related to density and size. This step is common for divide and conquer and stop and chop techniques of nucleus management.

In the author's opinion, a trench made properly can facilitate further steps of division, hold and chop, and nucleus management to a great extent. This chapter aims to discuss various aspects of trenching.

■ DEFINITION

Trench is sculpting of central hard part of nucleus—an important prerequisite for division of nucleus.

Parameters (Table 1): Phaco machine is to be set on phaco 1.

Energy:
- It is the most important parameter for trench.
- Energy should be both continuous and linear.
- Energy used should be adequate and based on density of nucleus.

For example,
- Hard nucleus needs more energy.
- Soft nucleus needs less energy.
- Energy variation also depends on sharpness of phaco tip.

Sharpness of phaco tip: For example, if you feel 70% energy for particular density of nucleus is required, then for sharp tip it may need 60% only, and for blunt tip it may need >70% of energy.

TABLE 1: Parameters.

Energy	Vacuum	Aspiration flow rate
60–70%	20–80 mm Hg	10–20 mm Hg

Vacuum and flow rates: They should be minimal as there is no specific role of these parameters during trench. But it is used to aspirate sculpted nuclear material which facilitates clear visualization for further trench.

Following discussion of trenching is with reference to stop and chop technique of nucleus management.

■ PREREQUISITE
Primary Position of Eyeball

Facilitates: Proper anatomical plane of trench and good red reflex can be visualised in immature cataract.

This primary position can be obtained by:
- Adjusting head position of patient by keeping chin and forehead parallel to floor before draping
- Bridle sutures for superior and inferior rectus
- Using chopper or fixation rod (Baile's eye lock) in side port
- Asking patient to look into the microscope light if procedure is under topical anesthesia

Optimum size of capsulorhexis, i.e., 4.5–5.5 mm, facilitates endo-capsular trenching, avoiding popping up of nucleus in anterior chamber (AC).

Immobile nucleus:
- It is the most important prerequisite in the author's opinion.
- *Immobility can be achieved by:*
  - Hydrodelineation (if possible)
  - Minimal or no hydrodissection
  - No rotation of nucleus before trench

■ TECHNIQUE
Checklist (Fig. 1)
- Check all parameters of phaco 1 by using a test chamber with phaco probe.
- Phaco tip (commonly used 30° tip and 45° Kelman tip) should be in *bevel up position with sideways irrigation.*

Trench

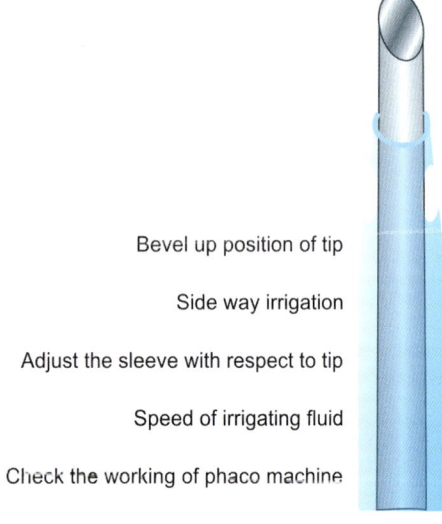

Bevel up position of tip
Side way irrigation
Adjust the sleeve with respect to tip
Speed of irrigating fluid
Check the working of phaco machine

Fig. 1: Checklist before start of trench.

- Adjust the sleeve with respect to phaco tip according to density of nucleus. It means soft nucleus needs small, exposed part of tip in front of the sleeve and large exposed part in hard nucleus.
- Check the speed of irrigating fluid and bottle height.
- Continuous irrigation should be on throughout the procedure.
- Set the energy according to density of nucleus based on preoperative assessment.
  - Pass phaco probe in bevel down or bevel horizontal position by slightly depressing posterior lip of incision.
  - Then rotate the tip into bevel up position.
  - Trench should be always in the central hard part of nucleus and usually within rhexis.
  - Depth and length of trench varies according to size and density of nucleus.
  - Start the trench at the superior border of capsulorhexis.

The first stroke should represent marking of trench and confirm its central location, if not then redirect next stroke in center only.

The second and third strokes of trench will give an idea about density and size of nucleus and energy parameters may be reset accordingly.

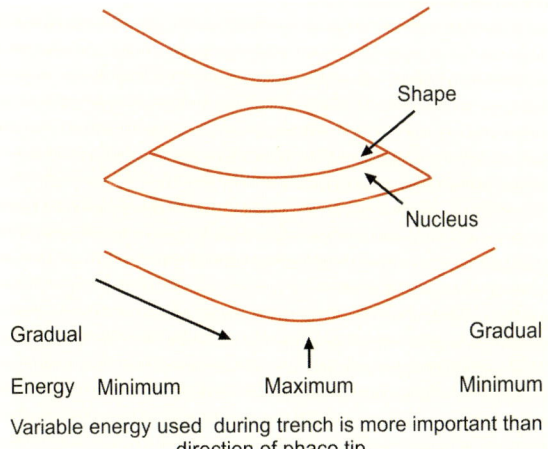

Fig. 2: Important points for consideration related to trench.

This is called feel of trench.
- Further strokes of the trench which are nearly parallel to the posterior capsule make the ideal shape of the trench.
- Ideal shape of trench should be shallow at both periphery and deep in the center **(Fig. 2)**.

WHAT THE IDEAL TRENCH IS?

- Central
- Narrow
- Usually within the capsulorhexis
- Uniplanar, i.e., single plane
- Deep in the center
- Depth should be half to two thirds of the hard part of the nucleus.
- Well-apposed steep walls

To achieve the abovementioned shape of trench (ideal trench), two factors are important **(Fig. 3)***:*
1. Direction of phaco probe which contributes only 30%
2. Most important factor is variable energy which contributes 70%. Energy should be minimum superiorly and increasing gradually toward center where it is maximum and then gradually decreases as you approach the inferior end.

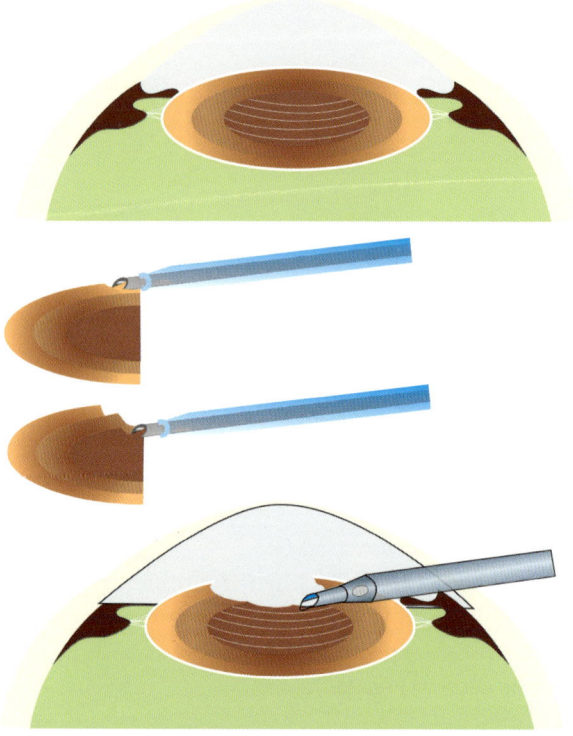

Trench should be done by lower one-third part of phaco tip

Fig. 3: Ideal design of trench.

- All strokes should be parallel to the posterior capsule.
- Trench should be done at *uniform speed*.
- Energy used during trench should be cut off while returning back.
- Angulation of phaco tip in such a way that lower one third of phaco tip should be used for sculpting the nucleus.
- With every stroke, one should shelve some layers of nucleus.

Some illustrations of trench are as follows:
- Trench is layer by layer sculpting of nucleus **(Fig. 4)**
  - Layer by layer sculpting is like cutting of wood by carpenter.
- Red reflex of groove varies with depth of trench **(Figs. 5A and B)**.
  - This is one of the important signs for depth of trench.

Trench

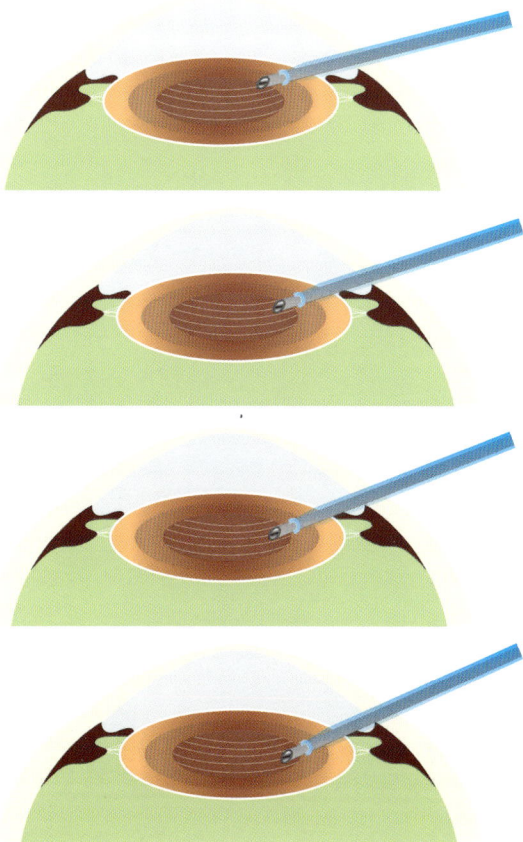

Fig. 4: Trench is layer-by-layer sculpting of nucleus.

- Correlation of phaco probe with incision **(Fig. 6)**
  - Straight phaco tip and Kelman tip behave in different ways related to incision.
- Trench by Kelman tip **(Figs. 7A and B)**
  - Does not affect the architecture of incision

Kelman tip with torsional technology:
- It works with Alcon Infiniti, Legion, and Centurion machine.
- It cuts the tissue by shearing force.
- *There is unique design of zigzag pattern in trench*—there is no pressure on zonules during trench.

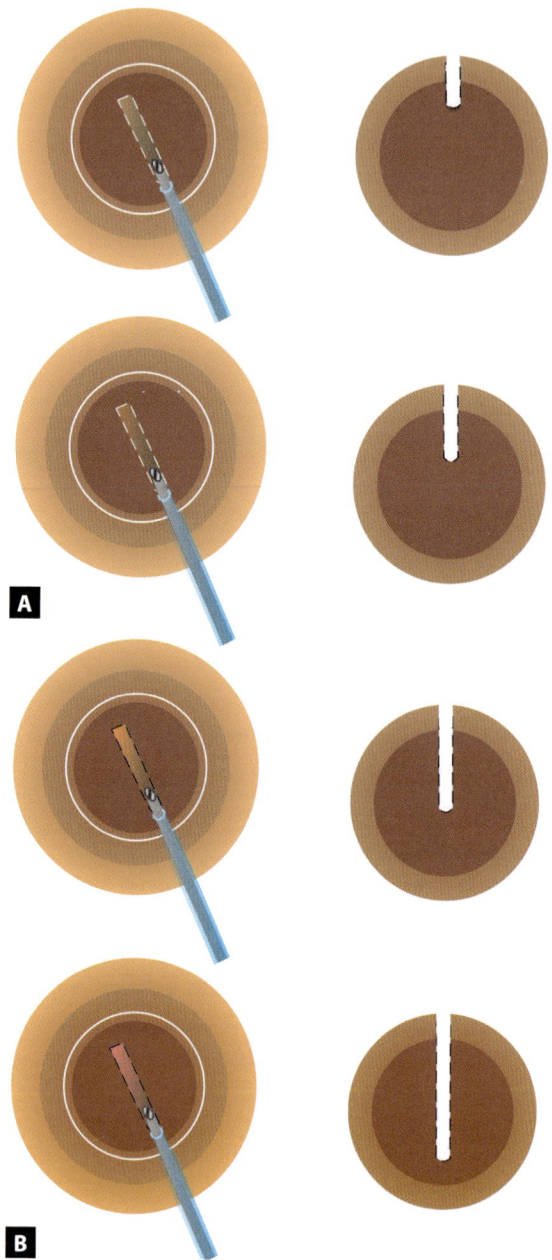

Figs. 5A and B: Red reflex of groove varies with depth of trench.

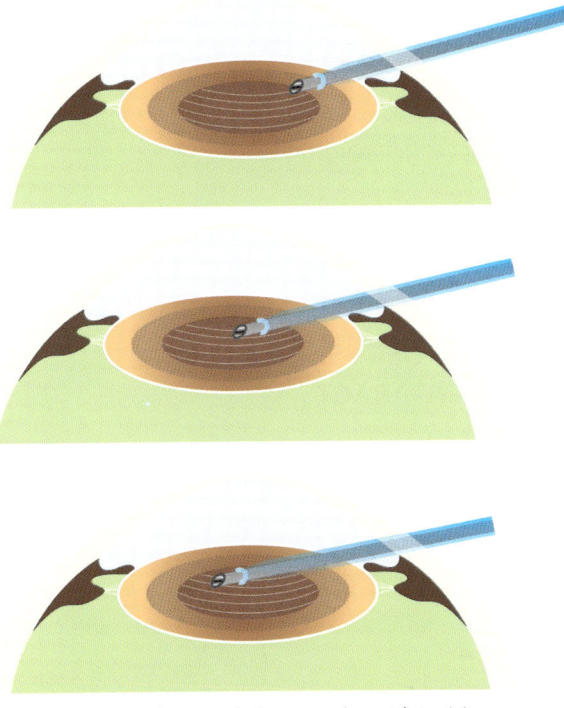

Fig. 6: Correlation of phaco probe with incision.

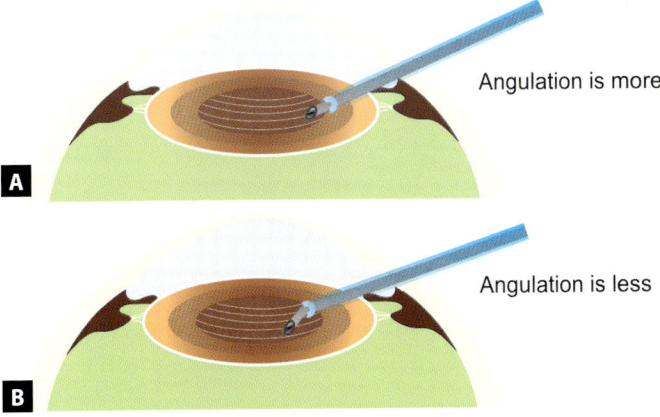

Figs. 7A and B: (A) With straight tip—more vertical stretching of the incision and (B) Kelman tip—avoid vertical stretching of the incision.

- Cases where one can suspect zonular weakness such as mature cataract, hard cataract, pseudexfoliation, and subluxated cataract—in these situations, trench by Kelman tip with torsional technology is safer.

Trench varies in the following ways:
- Shallow trench
- Long trench
- Deep inferiorly
- Shallow superiorly

VARIATIONS OF TRENCH IN DIFFERENT TYPES OF CATARACTS

Soft Cataract
- Less energy
- Shorter length related to the size of the nucleus
- Narrow
- Exposed part of tip in front of sleeve should be minimum.
- It is not necessary to go too deep in this situation.

Hard Cataract
- Exposed part of the tip in front of the sleeve should be more.
- Energy used should be more than normal parameters.
- Length and depth of trench usually more and will vary with hardness and size of nucleus
- Modified "funnel-shaped" trench is needed.
- Start trench as usual and after few strokes, start shelving of the anterior part of trench on both sides, i.e., anterior widening of superficial trench, so that sleeve will not get stuck in the walls of the trench during deep sculpting which is usually required in such cases.

White/Mature Cataract
- Density and size of nucleus are very variable and also unpredictable.
- After first few strokes, one should decide length and depth of trench accordingly.

Subluxated Cataract
- In cases where zonular weakness is found nasally or temporally
- Capsulorhexis is made away from weak zone—trench may be central or paracentral, i.e., away from zonular weakness area.
- Energy needed is more than adequate to avoid stress on zonules.
- Exposed part of tip in front of sleeve should be more to have adequate and fast sculpting of nucleus.

Shallow Anterior Chamber
- Shallow AC is usually associated with small pupil.
- Length of trench should be small.
- Energy used should be adequate or less as phaco probe is nearer to the cornea in these cases.
- Preferably, new tip should be used to minimize power requirement.
- Coating endothelium with dispersive viscoelastics can give additional protection to endothelium in these cases.
- First stroke should be horizontal, then bevel up position for further strokes of trench.

Pseudoexfoliation Cataract
- It is usually associated with a poorly dilating pupil, i.e., small pupil.
- Capsulorhexis should be made within border of pseudoexfoliated material and hence:
  - Capsulorhexis should be small and thus, trench should be small in length.
  - Energy used should be more than adequate to avoid stress on the zonules which is already compromised.

Cataract in Vitrectomized Eyes
Energy used for trench should be more than adequate so that with minimum strokes, adequate depth can be achieved.

Cataract with High Myopia
- In these cases, cataracts may be soft or hard. There may be compromised zonules, hypotony and deep AC.
- Energy used should be more than adequate and trench will be according to density of nucleus.

Small Pupil

Trench should be small in length.

Hazy Cornea

- Dispersive viscoelastics used for protection of endothelium
- Relatively small capsulorhexis is required which ensures protection of the cornea as energy during the trench in peripheral zone will be cut off by anterior capsule.

■ COMPLICATIONS OF TRENCH

- During the trench, the surgeon may catch the iris or cut anterior capsule.
- Due to more manipulation, i.e., more strokes of trench pupil may get smaller.
- Sometimes due to inadequate energy, there is a stress on zonules and zonular dehiscence can occur due to mechanical pressure on lens.
- *Air bubbles formation into the AC:*
    - Due to more energy used during trench than needed
    - Air bubbles enter via irrigation line
    - Collision between water current and viscoelastics in AC
- Posterior capsule rupture can occur usually in inferior part of trench.
- Corneal haze or burn
- Distortion of main incision.

■ FACTORS NEEDED TO MASTER THIS IMPORTANT STEP OF PHACO

- Synchronization between foot pedal and phaco probe
- Assessment of the depth of the trench
- Maintenance of the uniform speed of phaco tip
- Energy used with respect to particular size and density of nucleus
- Energy used for particular site of the nucleus which means variable energy used for different zones, such as periphery, midperiphery and center.

VARIATIONS IN DESIGN OF TRENCH DURING LEARNING PHASE (FIG. 8) AND TRENCH RELATED TO DIFFERENT MINDSET (FIG. 9)

It is very important to achieve the ideal trench. After studying various trenches of different surgeons, the author has put this new concept

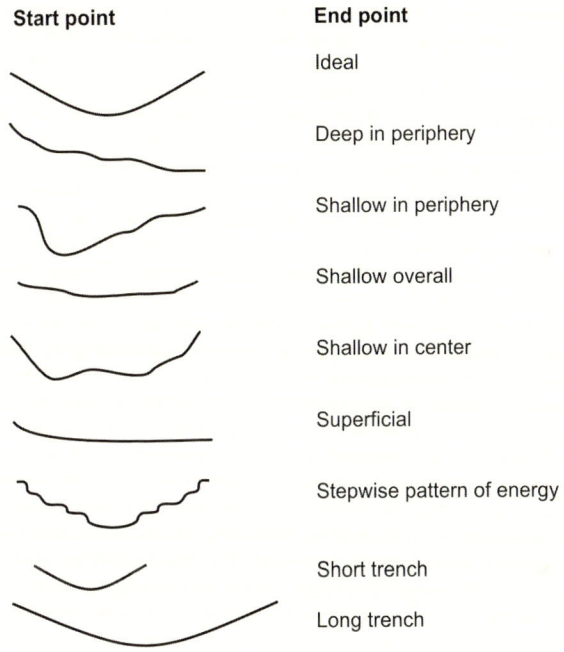

Fig. 8: Variation in designs of trench during learning phase.

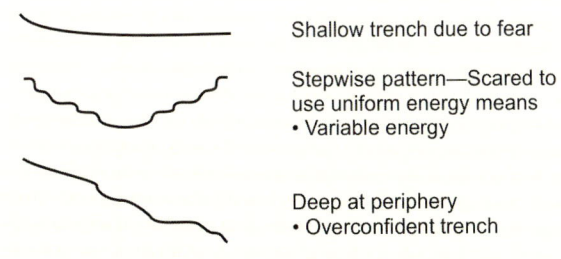

Fig. 9: Trench related to different mindset.

of variation in design of trench and its relationship with different mindset for better analysis of groove and its significance for further procedure.

■ KEY POINTS

- It is the most important step in nucleus management.
- Trench should be central, narrow, usually within capsulorhexis, uniplanar, deep in center, and half to two-thirds deep, well-apposed steep walls.
- Immobile nucleus is the most important prerequisite for trench which can be achieved by minimal or no hydroprocedures and no rotation of nucleus before trench.
- Ideal trench is helpful for division of nucleus.

■ LIVE SURGERY PHOTOGRAPHS (FIGS. 10A TO M)

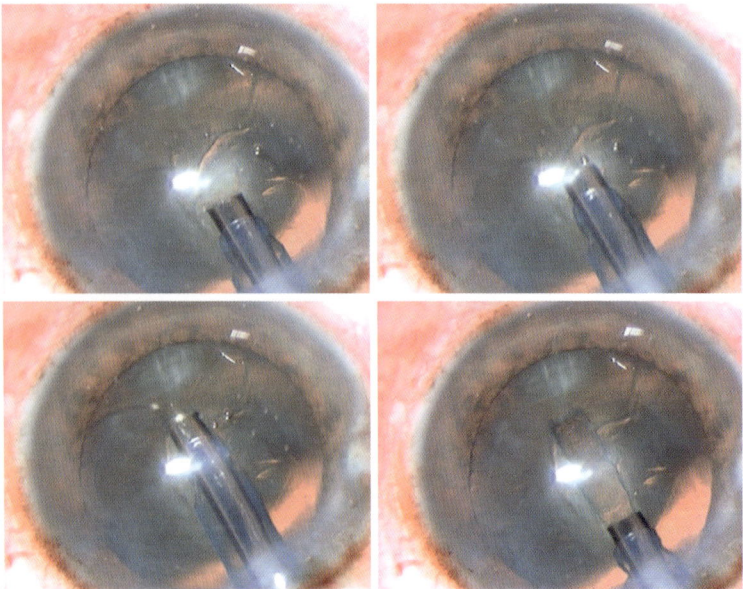

Fig. 10A: Trench on immobile nucleus (no rotation of nucleus before trench).

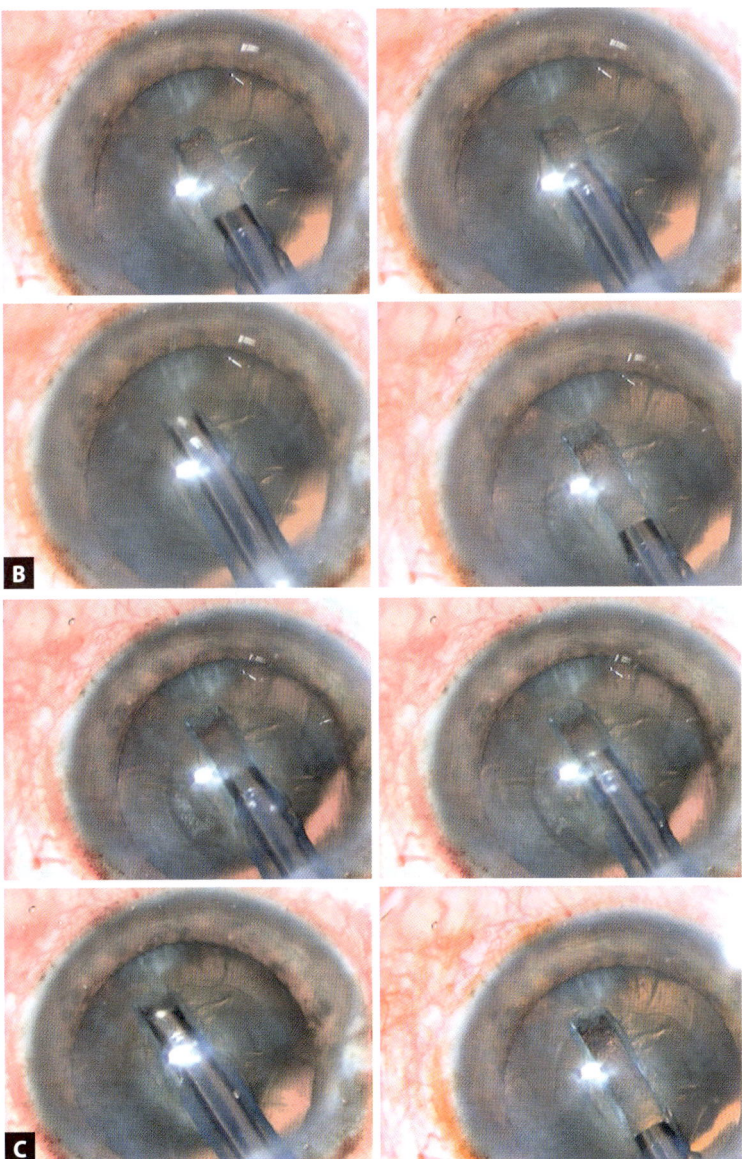

Figs. 10B and C: (B) Such trench is always stable; (C) Trench is central, narrow within capsulorhexis and with well-apposed walls.

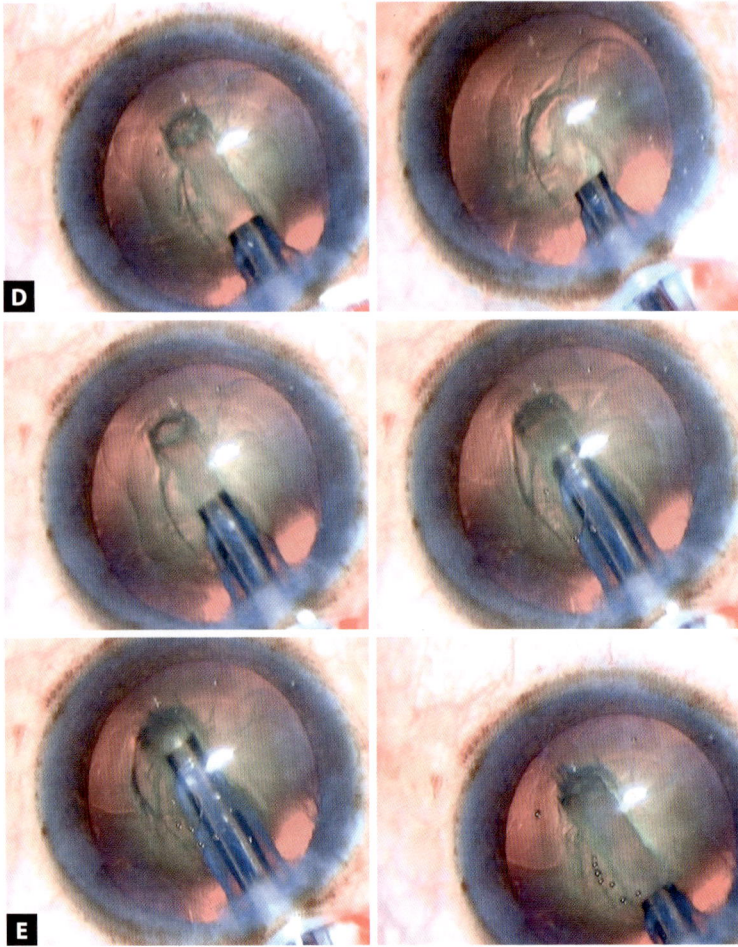

Figs. 10D and E: (D) Trench on immobile nucleus (no hydro before trench). Water waves seen during trench; (E) In trench, energy should be used maximum to preset values.

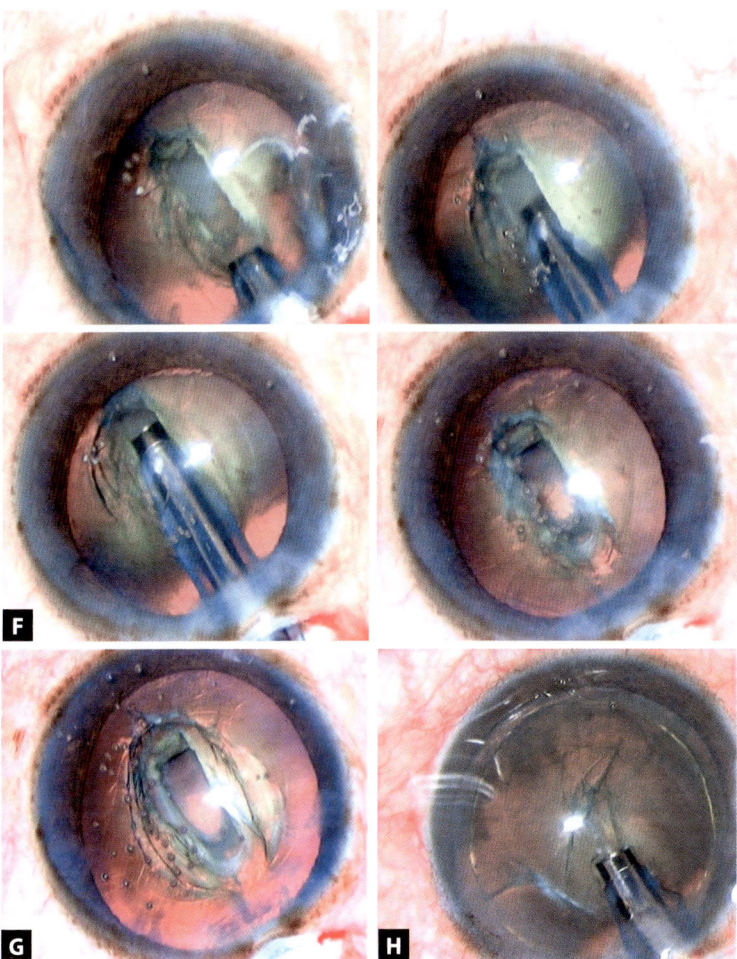

Figs. 10F to H: (F) Trench is adequately deep—means half to two-thirds of nucleus thickness with central red reflex; (G) Final result of an ideal trench means central, narrow, within capsulorhexis, not too long, deep enough, and most importantly, with well-apposed walls which is a prerequisite for division; (H) Phaco tip bevel up position to start trench.

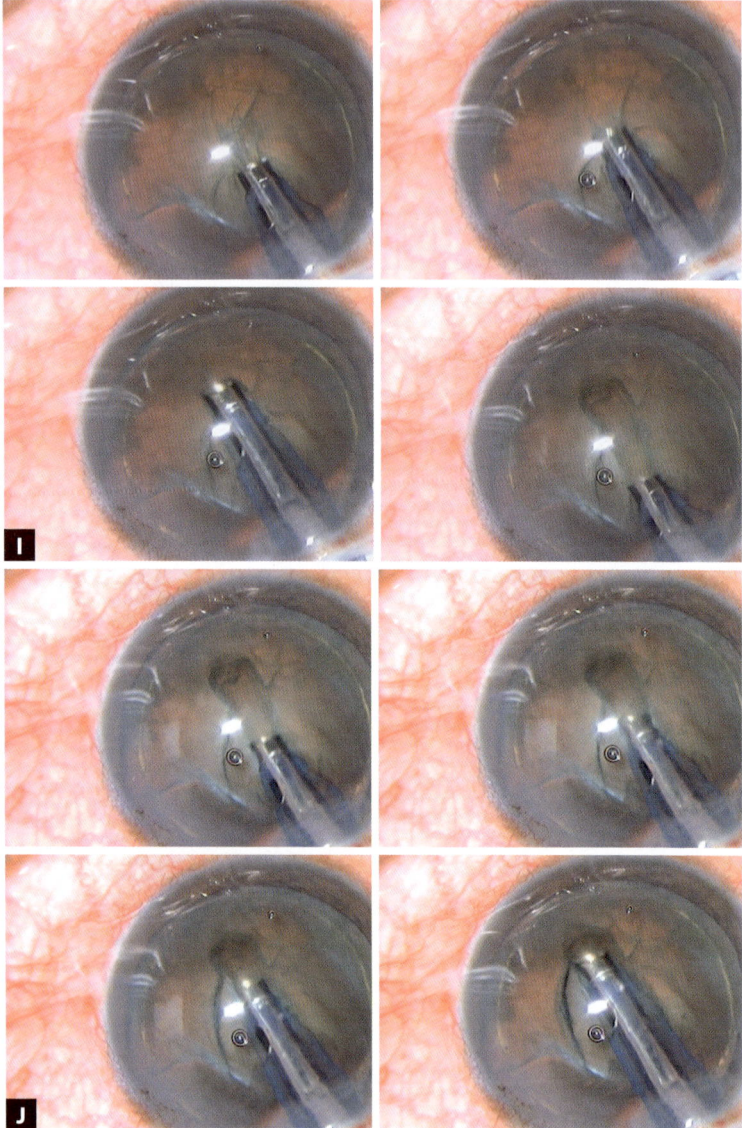

Figs. 10I and J: (I) Trench should be superficial. First stroke of trench is for marking the center; (J) Second stroke of trench will give an idea about consistency of the nucleus.

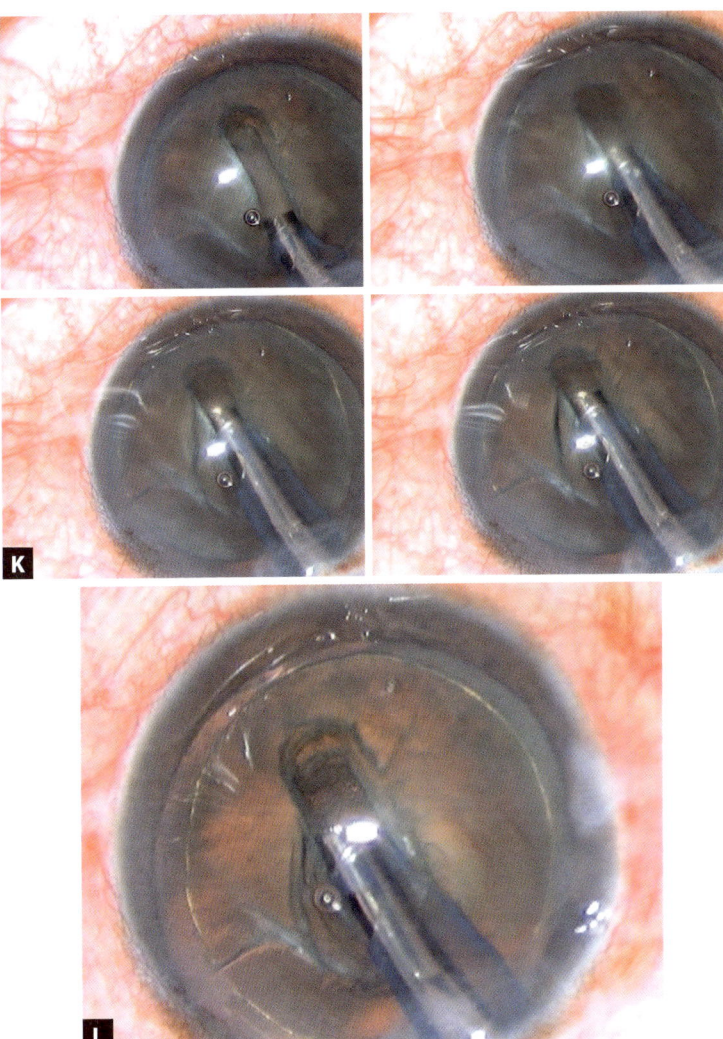

Figs. 10K and L: (K) Trench should always be layer-by-layer deepening of the central hard part of nucleus; (L) While coming back, no energy should be used—foot pedal position one or two.

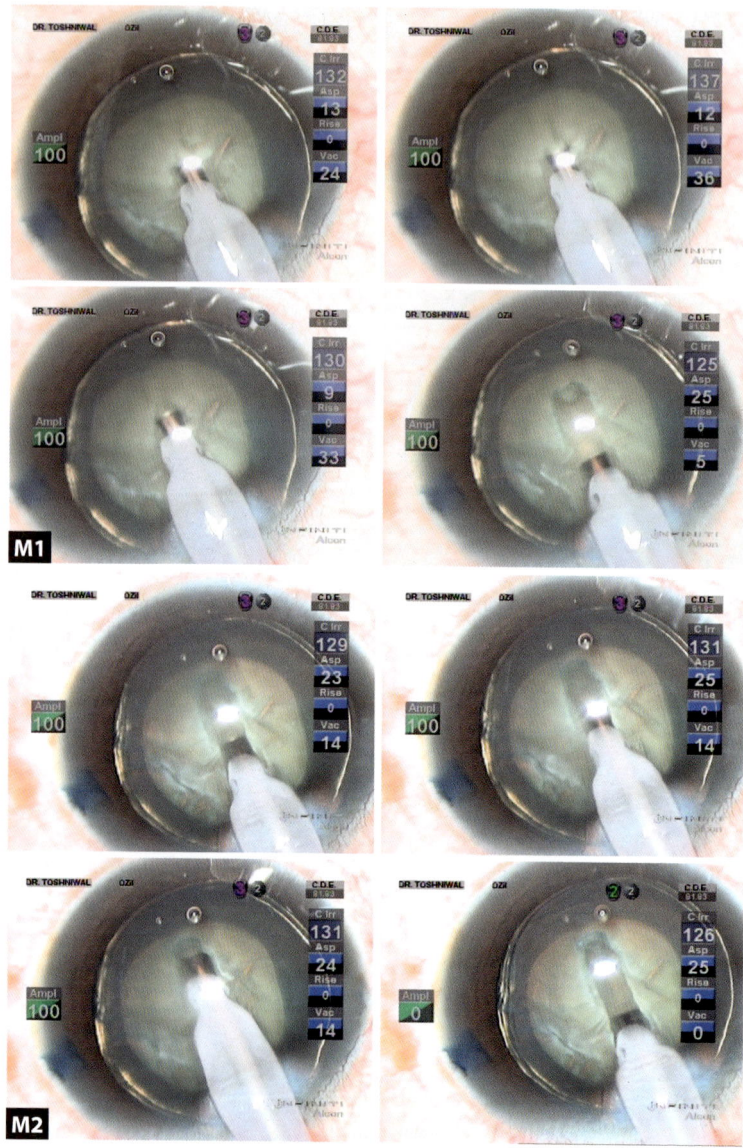

Figs. 10M1 and M2: (M1) Trench by Kelman tip with torsional phaco technology; (M2) Central superficial trench.

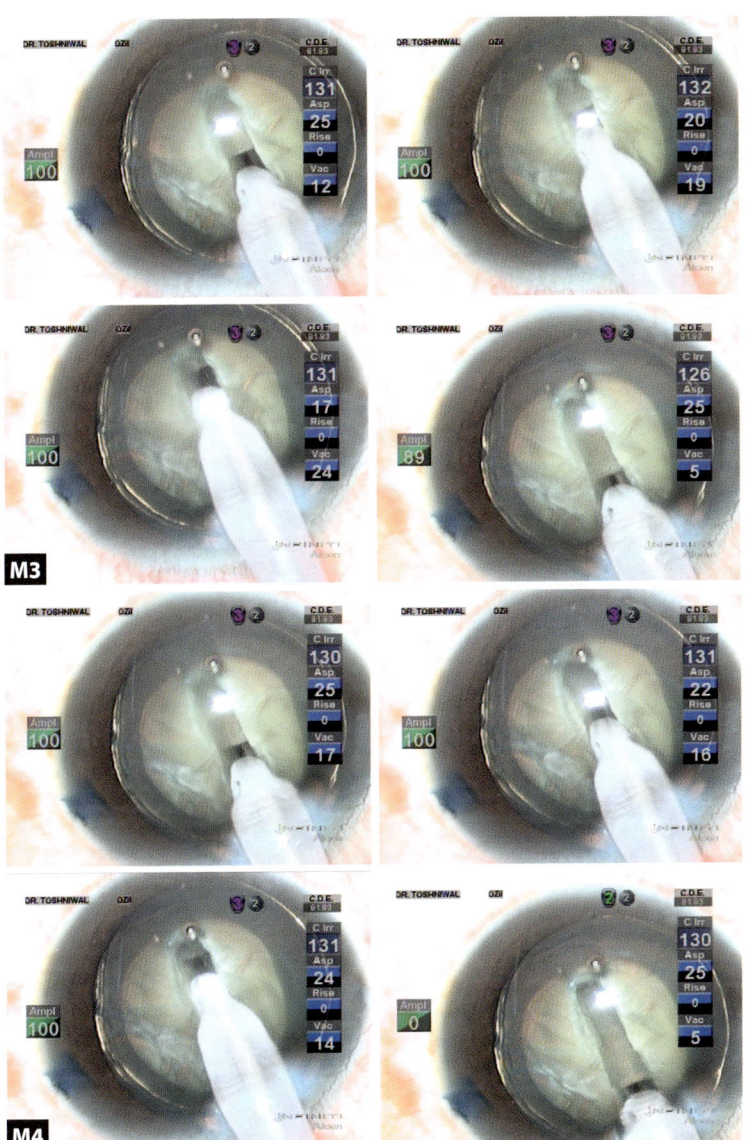

Figs. 10M3 and M4: (M3) Trench layer-by-layer; (M4) Apposition of Kelman tip to nucleus tissue is easy because of design of the tip.

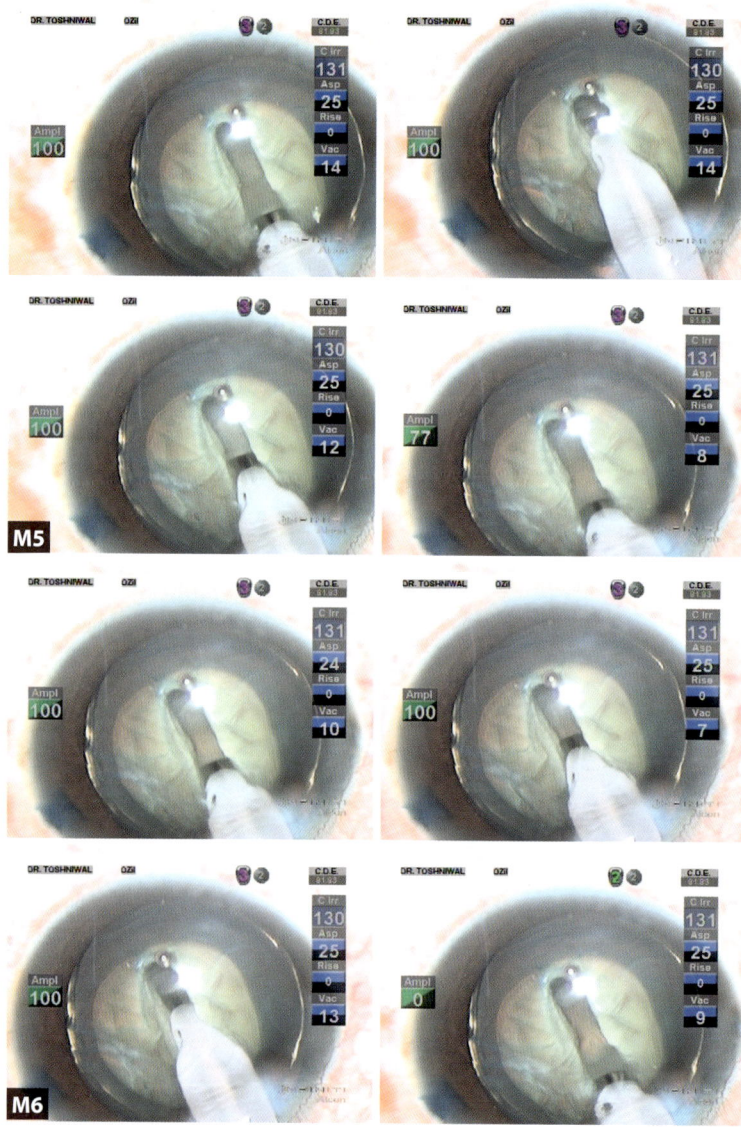

Figs. 10M5 and M6: (M5) Another advantage of Kelman tip: As the trench goes deeper and deeper, still there is no vertical stretching of wound; (M6) Finally, ideal trench with perfect centration, related to golden ring.

CHAPTER 10

Division of Nucleus

■ INTRODUCTION

Division of nucleus is the procedure performed after trench which provides two halves of equal sizes or nearly equal sizes of nucleus.

Ideal trench is the most important prerequisite for good division.

Good division provides the surgeon with a flat surface in each nuclear hemisphere where one can hold the nucleus halves adequately and chop accordingly.

It is one of the most crucial steps in stop and chop technique of phacoemulsification in the sense that even after an ideal trench, many surgeons have difficulty in performing complete division of the nucleus.

This chapter highlights the detailed procedure of ideal division of the nucleus.

■ PREREQUISITE

- *Ideal trench:* It will help in dividing the nucleus into two equal halves.
- *Visualization of the base of the trench:* It helps in proper placement of instruments needed for division.
- *Primary position of the eyeball:* It gives better visualization of the groove of the trench and helps to do the procedure of division in an ideal way.
- Adequate anterior chamber depth
- *Nucleus bulk:* The bulk of nucleus is required so that one can apply force to get the ideal division.

■ PRINCIPLE (FIG. 1)

- Divide the nucleus in central hard part
- Equal force needed to divide the nucleus
- Force should be parallel to each other.

Division of Nucleus

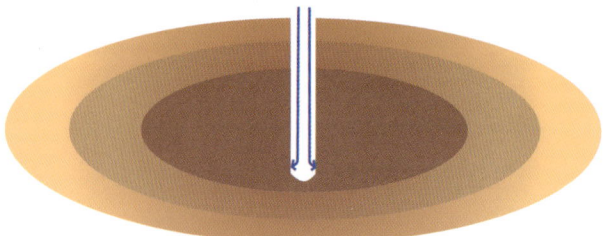

Fig. 1: Principle of division: Division should be in the central hard part of nucleus; equal pressure on each half of nucleus; and direction of division should be in a single plane.

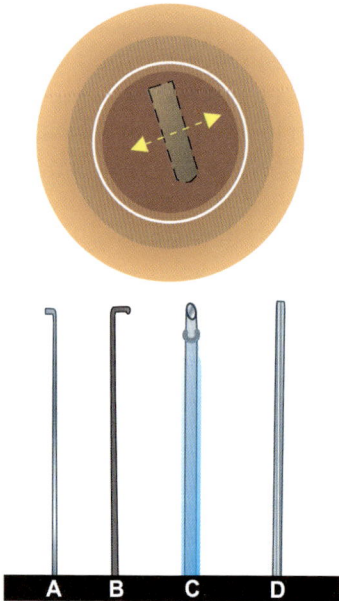

Figs. 2A to D: Basic instruments used for division: (A) Dialer; (B) Chopper; (C) Phaco tip; and (D) Viscocannula.

Basic Instruments Used for Division (Figs. 2A to D)

- Dialer
- Chopper
- Phaco tip
- Viscocannula

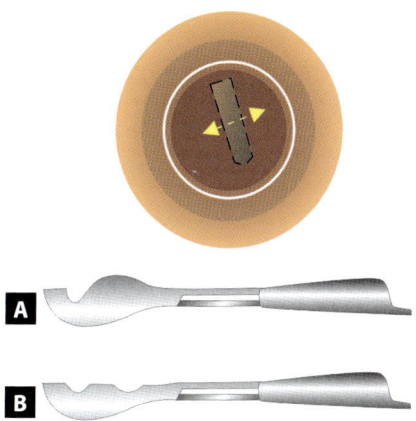

Figs. 3A and B: Special instruments used for division: (A) Akahoshi prechopper and (B) Toshniwal prechopper.

Special Instruments Used for Division (Figs. 3A and B)
- Akahoshi prechopper
- Toshniwal prechopper

■ TECHNIQUES (FIGS. 4A TO E) (TABLE 1)
Procedure

Division with the help of a dialer and a chopper is the preferred two-handed technique by the author. First, the anterior chamber should be filled with viscoelastics and at the same time, the surgeon pushes the visco also near the trench to get a good view at its base. The surgeon has to assess whether the trench is of adequate size, depth, and architecture and then only one should proceed with the division of the nucleus. After careful assessment, the surgeon then passes the chopper from the side port. Then the dialer is inserted from the main port incision to reach the center of the nucleus which is the main bulk of nucleus. Now, the division is tried by giving equal and simultaneous forces by both instruments at one plane, parallel to each other but in opposite direction, i.e., the chopper should give the force toward the left side and at the same time the dialer should give an equal force toward the right side. These maneuvers are to be done ideally at the deepest part of the trench or at the junction of the

Division of Nucleus

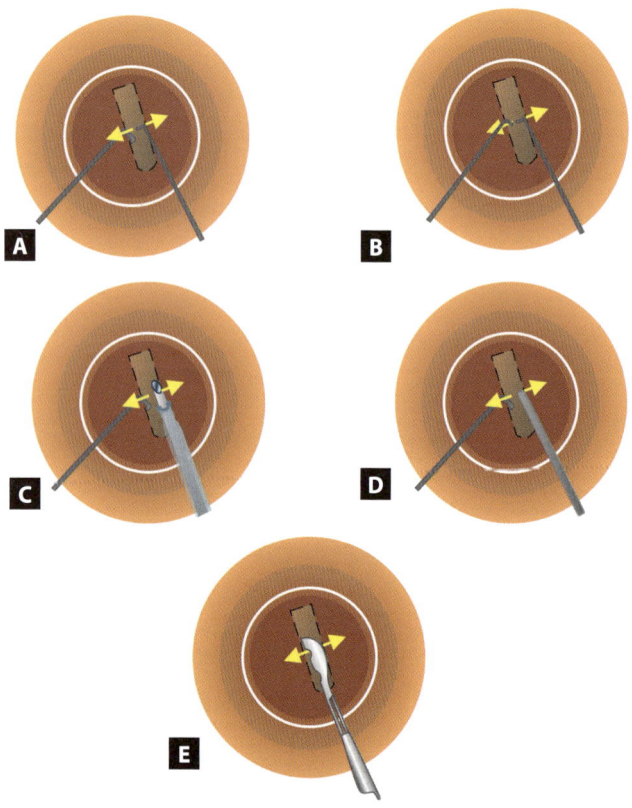

Figs. 4A to E: Different techniques of nucleus division. (A) Dialer and chopper; (B) Dialer and dialer; (C) Phaco tip and chopper; (D) Viscocannula and chopper for confirmation of division; and (E) Toshniwal prechopper.

TABLE 1: Instruments used for division.

In the right hand	In the left hand	Types of technique
Dialer	Chopper	Two-handed technique
Dialer	Dialer	Two-handed technique
Phaco tip	Chopper	Two-handed technique
Viscocannula	Chopper	Two-handed technique for confirmation of division
Prechopper		One-handed technique

anterior two thirds and the posterior one third of the nucleus bulk. During this procedure, excessive force or pressure to the cornea or zonules should be avoided. If done at a correct plane with an ideal trench with correct principles in mind, one can divide by simple use of little force which will never distort the cornea or give any pressure to the zonules. Sometimes, the surgeon may stabilize the left-side piece with the help of the chopper and then use dialer to give the force on the opposite piece and get the central division.

Thus, with this procedure, a surgeon will always be able to get a clear central division, following which surgeon needs to confirm that the division is complete. This is one of the most important step as without this step the hold and lift of the nucleus piece is not possible. To do this, the surgeon should use the viscocannula in his right hand and insert it in the anterior chamber from the main port-incision and fill the anterior chamber with the visco and again inject the visco to visualize the complete division.

If division is not complete, the tip of the canula which is passed through the main port and the chopper through left side port are placed at the base where division has not occurred and where equal and opposite forces are applied at the respective halves of the nucleus for complete division, and one can see a good red glow between the two halves of the nucleus.

Throughout this procedure, the anterior chamber is well maintained by viscoelastics, which is having an advantage of better visualization throughout the procedure and at the same time to repeat the same maneuver to detach the strands of nuclear fibers at different points.

Finally with a gentle force at the edge of the hard part of the nucleus, one can easily rotate the nucleus halves to the desired position for hold and lift.

Ideal Division (Fig. 5)

Division should be in the center, which results in two equal hemispheres of nucleus.

Division with Dialer and Chopper

Advantages:
- Two instruments of equal size usually give equal force for division.

Division of Nucleus

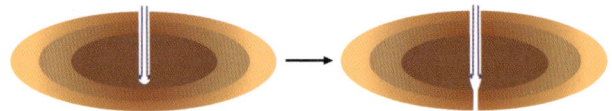

Fig. 5: Ideal division.

- Two thin instruments can be easily placed through a narrow groove.
- Two instruments can easily reach the base of the trench at the desired level.
- With these two instruments, peripheral division of the inferior tags of the nucleus can be easily done, and it is even more significant for releasing the superior tags too.
- Many times, division of the nucleus and at the same time rotation of the two halves of the nucleus can be easily possible at the desired position for further hold and chop.
- Easy to perform

Disadvantages:
- Repeated passing of these instruments in and out is needed.
- Anterior chamber collapses during this maneuver, so one should maintain the anterior chamber by putting viscoelastics repeatedly.
- It is an additional step because once the division is made by the phaco tip and the chopper, you may proceed to the next step of nucleus management immediately.
- Damage to the cornea, iris, and anterior capsule can be possible as both instruments are sharp.

Division with Phaco Tip and Chopper

Advantages:
- Since the phaco tip is used which has a continuous irrigation, the anterior chamber depth is always maintained.
- One can finish the trench and directly go for the division step without other instrumentation; therefore, the surgical time is reduced.
- Visualization is better all the time as one can use aspiration to clear away any loose cortex that is present at the base of the

trench or surrounding area which hinders the visualization of the surgeon.
- Mild rotation of the nucleus halves, which is required sometimes to get to the desired position of hold and chop, can be performed very easily.
- Phaco probe is introduced only once and does not disrupt the architecture of the main port incision.

Disadvantages:
- Since unequal forces are applied, one gets unequal division of nucleus with one large and other small piece.
- There are chances of iris coming out of the incision.
- Partial division of the nucleus can occur more frequently.
- Attached superior tags are difficult to detach, as the phaco tip cannot easily reach the desired position superiorly.

■ AKAHOSHI PRECHOPPER

Akahoshi Prechopper—introduced by Dr Akahoshi (Japan) for division of nucleus without trench but the author used this instrument for division after trench of nucleus.

■ TOSHNIWAL PRECHOPPER (FIG. 6)

- Lightweight
- Blunt from all sides
- Passes through 2.00 mm incision
- When placed vertically, anterior surface has two notches for better visibility of groove of trench and depth of trench. Posterior surface is curved to place the instrument parallel to posterior capsule before division.

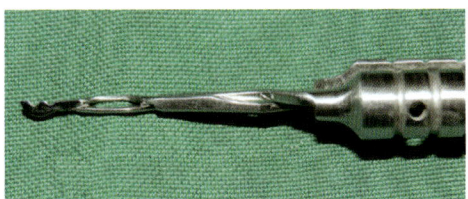

Fig. 6: Toshniwal prechopper.

■ PROCEDURE (FIG. 7)

Placement of Toshniwal prechopper is illustrated in **Figure 7**.
Advantages:
- This is a one-handed technique; thus, more effective and easier workup can be done by the surgeon.
- The instrument provides equal forces, with broader plates (thus increasing the area of contact between the instrument and

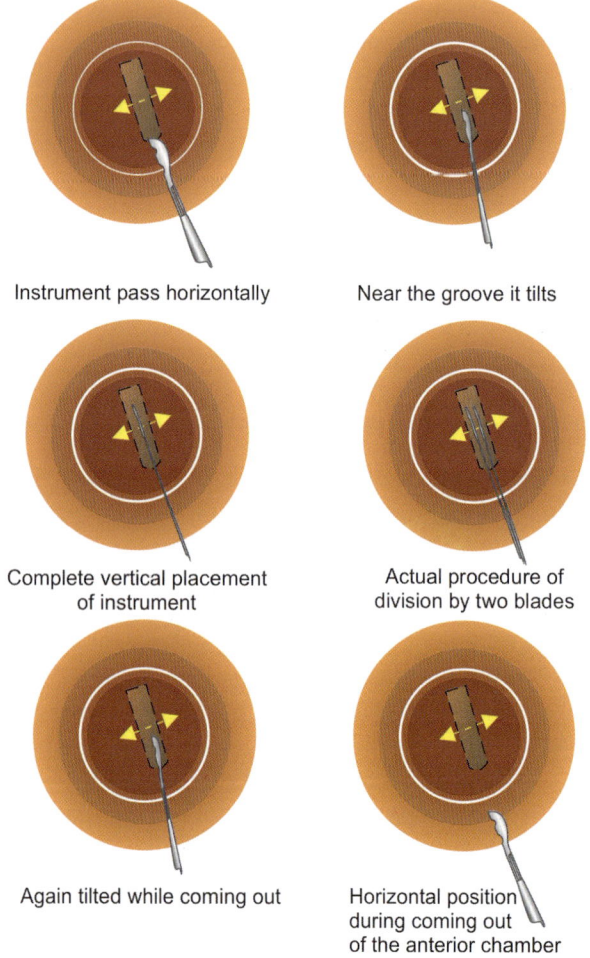

Fig. 7: Division by Toshniwal prechopper.

nucleus), which works perfectly at parallel planes to each other and always in opposite direction to each other and therefore, there is nearly equal division.
- Since all the principles of division work at their level best with simplicity, damage to the bag and the zonules is reduced.
- This prechopper has flat plates; thus, the force is at a wider area as compared to the chopper and dialer, so the chances of this instrument going inside the soft nucleus of a soft cataract during division is nearly absent, so division is easy in a soft cataract.
- Since this instrument gives least pressure on the zonules and the bag, this instrument is considered as the instrument of choice for the division in cases with suspicious weak bag and zonules, such as pseudoexfoliation, mature cataract, hard cataract, and subluxated cataract.
- Forces applied are always at the center of the nucleus, so the division is always near to perfect.
- One can repeat the procedure of division several times to check completion of division.

Disadvantages:
- The chamber usually gets collapsed with attempt of division, so one has to refill the anterior chamber with visco and then only can one reuse this instrument to do further division or for the confirmation of the division.
- This is one of the costly instruments in ophthalmic surgical practice.

IMPORTANT TIPS RELATED TO DIVISION (FIGS. 8A TO C)

Correlation of force, site, and direction for division is demonstrated and direction of division in hard nucleus is also illustrated in **Figures 8A to C**.

DIFFERENT HAPPENINGS DURING DIVISION (FIGS. 9A TO C)

During division, sometimes plane and pressure vary from case to case.

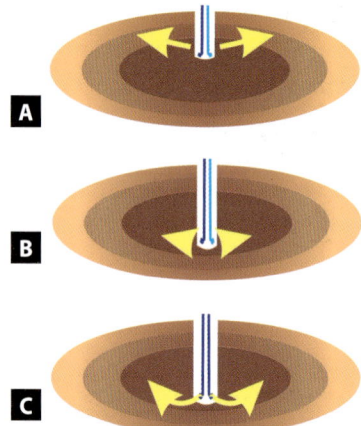

Figs. 8A to C: Important tips related to division: (A) More pressure is needed to divide in superficial groove; (B) Less pressure needed to divide deep trench; and (C) Direction of pressure needed to divide hard nucleus.

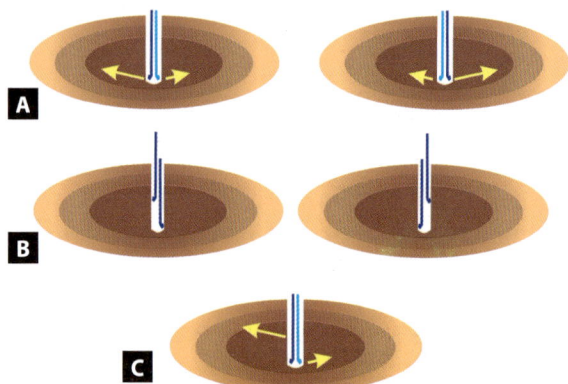

Figs. 9A to C: Different happenings during division: (A) Same plane but unequal pressure; (B) Same pressure but unequal plane; and (C) Unequal plane and unequal pressure.

■ CORRELATION OF TRENCH WITH DIVISION

- Different depth in trench **(Figs. 10A1 to A4)**
- Variation in groove with respect to width **(Figs. 10B1 and B2)**

Division of Nucleus

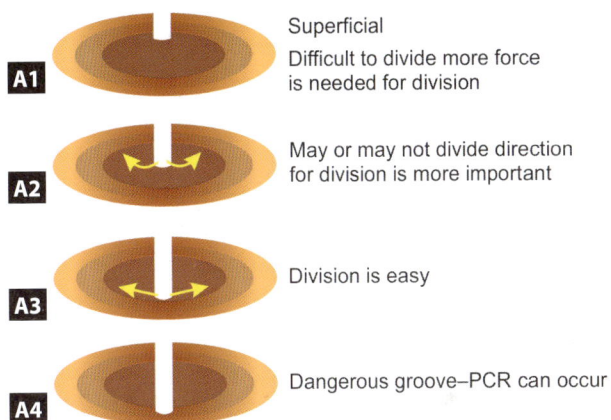

Figs. 10A1 to A4: Correlation of trench with division. Different depth in trench: (A1) Less than half the depth of nucleus; (A2) Half the depth of nucleus; (A3) Two-thirds or more than two-thirds depth of nucleus; and (A4) Very deep trench.

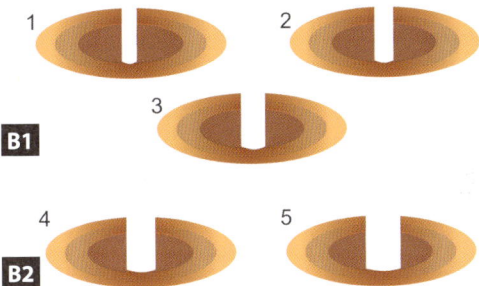

Figs. 10B1 and B2: Correlation of trench with division. Variation in groove with respect to width: (B1) Easy to divide in situations 1, 2, and 3 and (B2) difficult to divide in situations 4 and 5.

- *Unequal groove:* Difficult to divide and further nucleus management **(Fig. 10C)**

■ DIVISION IN SOFT CATARACT (FIGS. 11A AND B)

Flat surface of blades of Toshniwal prechopper hastens division.

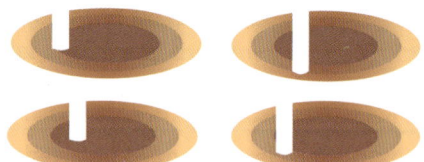

Fig. 10C: Correlation of trench with division. Unequal grooves—difficult to divide and further nucleus management.

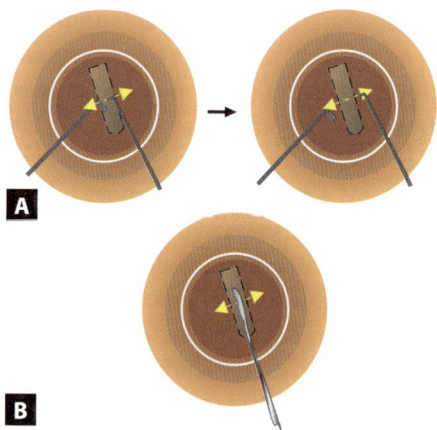

Figs. 11A and B: Division in soft cataract: (A) Difficult to divide with dialer and chopper as these two sharp instruments are passing through the substance of soft nucleus without effective division; (B) With the help of prechopper, division can be possible in soft cataract as plates are working for division.

▪ COMPLICATIONS OF DIVISION

- Shallowing of the anterior chamber which may cause damage to the anterior and posterior capsules, iris, and cornea.
- Zonular dialysis
- Posterior capsular rent at the periphery

▪ DIFFICULTIES DURING DIVISION

- Concentration on two instruments with synchronization of manipulation, with the two-handed technique.
- Excessive pressure of instruments on the incision sites
- Shallowing of the anterior chamber
- Displacement of the eyeball

- Difficulties related to anatomy of the lens, for example, soft cataract, sticky cataract, hard cataract, dense posterior subcapsular cataract, preexisting shallow anterior chamber, and small pupil.

■ KEY POINTS
- Division is the most crucial step and needs more practice.
- Ideal division is important for hold and chop of each half of nucleus.
- Toshniwal prechopper—changed scenario of this step and made it simpler and easier.

■ LIVE SURGERY PHOTOGRAPHS (FIGS. 12A TO P)

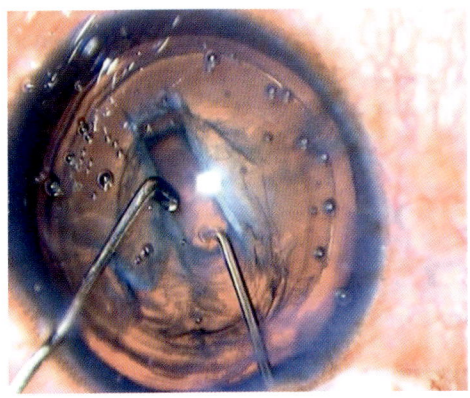

Fig. 12A: Dialer through main port and chopper via side port is ideal for division.

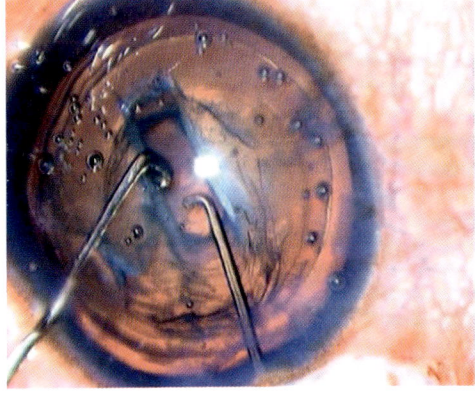

Fig. 12B: Two equal size and weight instruments usually divide the nucleus in two equal halves.

Division of Nucleus

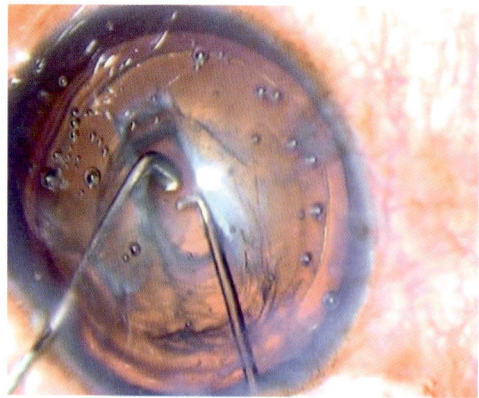

Fig. 12C: Two instruments placed deep in the center of the trench.

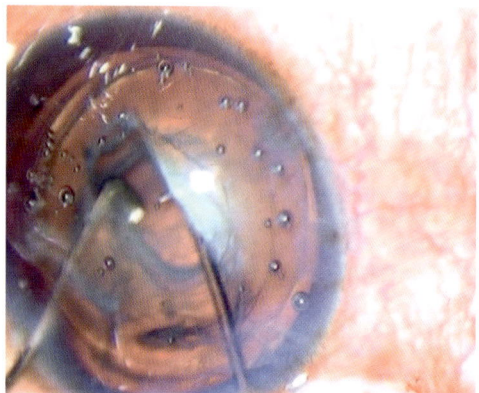

Fig. 12D: Two instruments move in opposite direction with equal force and at one plane.

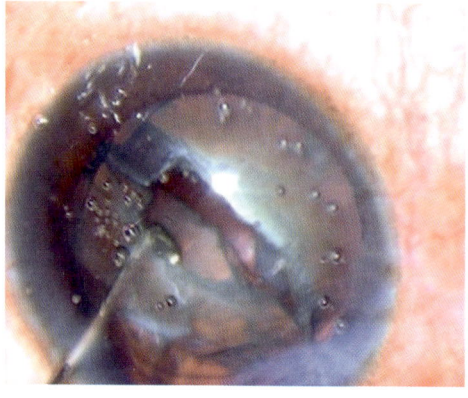

Fig. 12E1

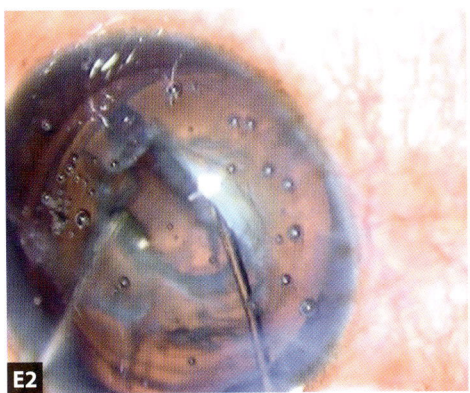

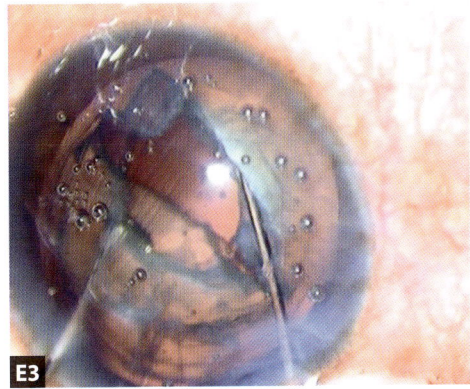

Figs. 12E2 and E3
Figs. 12E1 to E3: Division started and completed.

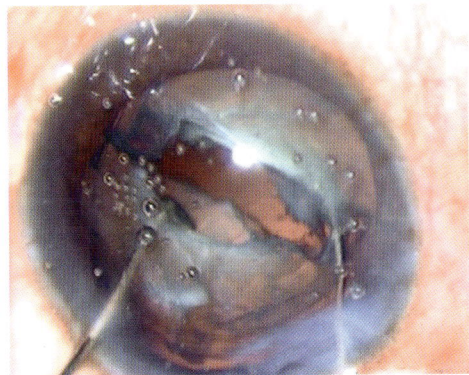

Fig. 12F1

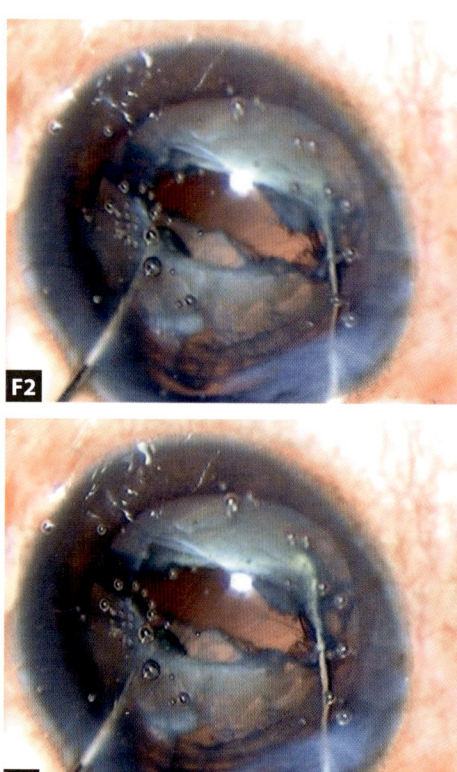

Figs. 12F2 and F3
Figs. 12F1 to F3: Placement of the instrument at the periphery for rotation.

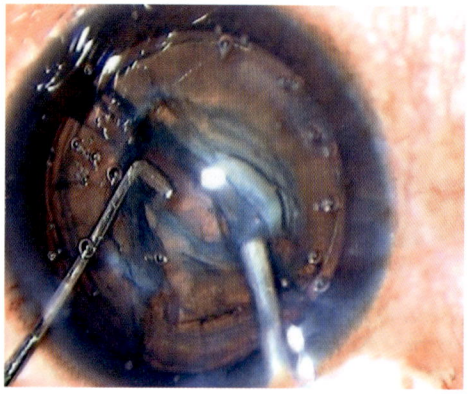

Fig. 12G: Viscocannula introduced via main port to confirm the division by injecting the visco in the gap of division.

Division of Nucleus

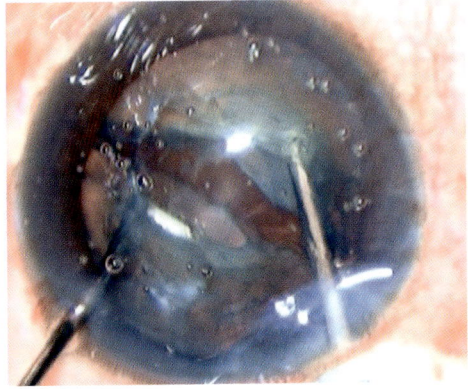

Fig. 12H: Confirmation of division and rotation is done by viscocannula and chopper while maintaining the anterior chamber.

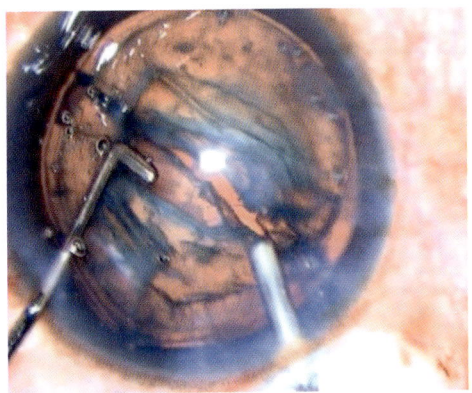

Fig. 12I: Finally, complete division occurred, and piece is ready for hold and chop.

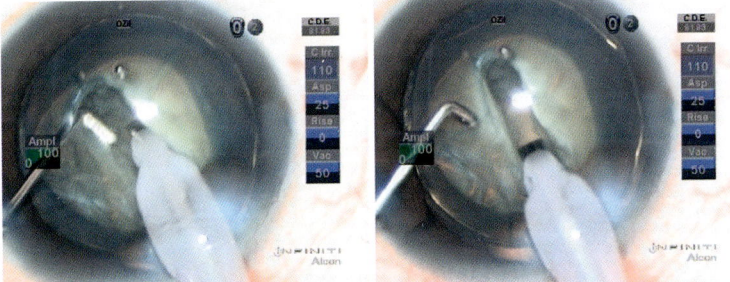

Fig. 12J: Phaco tip and chopper are used for division.

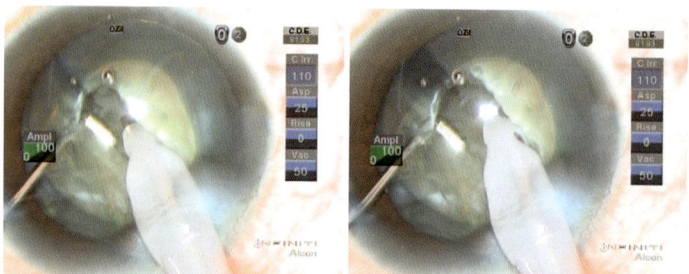

Fig. 12K: Principle applied for division is same. The advantage is that anterior chamber is maintained.

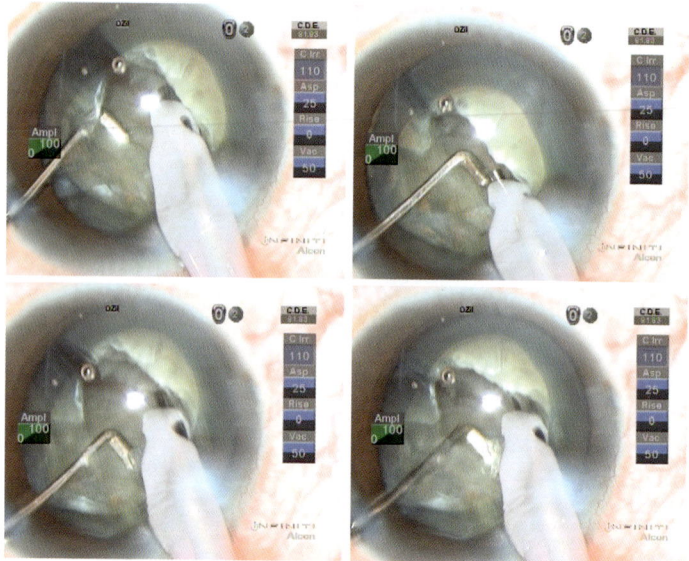

Fig. 12L: Division completed and nucleus rotation started.

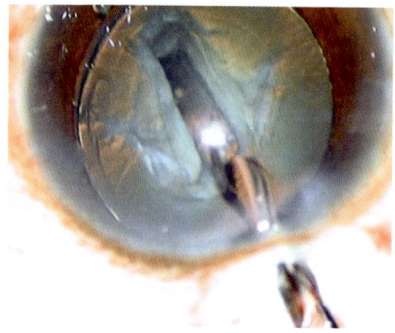

Fig. 12M: Prechopper introduced.

Division of Nucleus

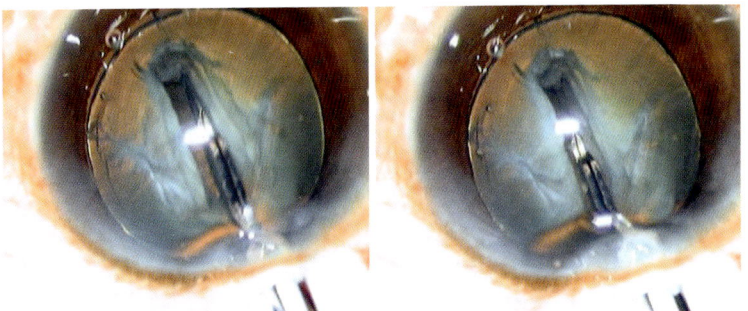

Fig. 12N: Placement of the prechopper deep in the center of the groove.

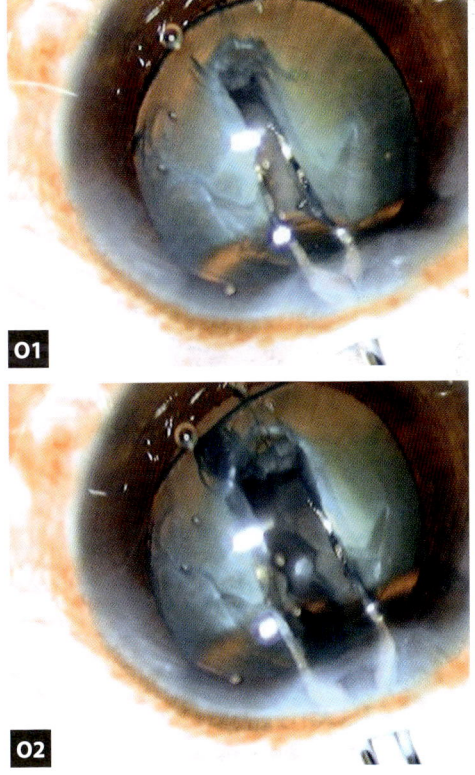

Figs. 12O1 and O2

Division of Nucleus

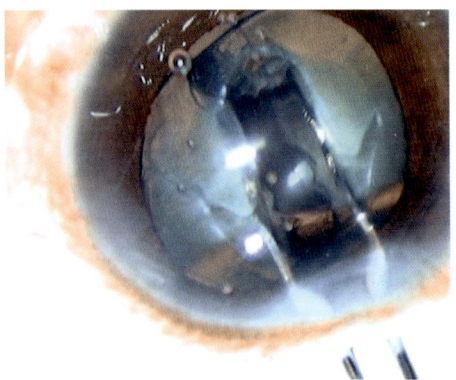

Fig. 12O3
Figs. 12O1 to O3: Division started and completed.

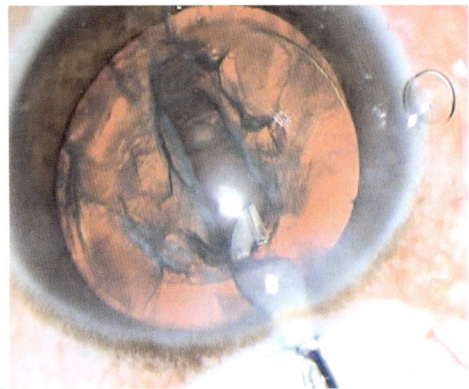

Fig. 12P: Horizontal placement of prechopper for going in and coming out of the eye.

CHAPTER 11
Hold and Chop of Nucleus

■ INTRODUCTION

In stop and chop technique, after trench and division, hold and chop of each hemisphere of nucleus is to be done. Hold and chop is a conceptual step in phaco surgery. After a good hold and chopping of the pieces, removal of the nuclear pieces is easy.

■ INSTRUMENTS NEEDED (FIGS. 1A AND B)
- Phaco tip for hold
- Chopper for chopping

Designs of the Phaco Tip (Fig. 2)

Phaco tip is designed from 0° to 60° tip. Hold and cutting of nucleus depends on angulation. Cutting efficiency is more with more angulation.

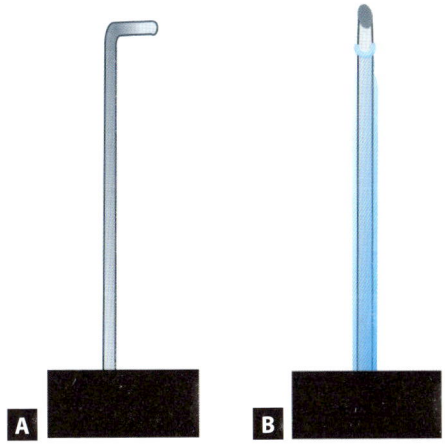

Figs. 1A and B: Instruments needed for hold and chop: (A) Chopper and (B) Phaco tip.

Hold and Chop of Nucleus

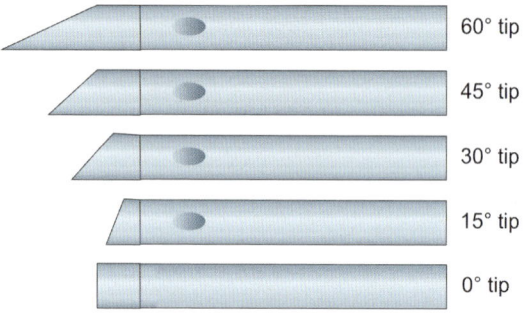

Fig. 2: Designs of the phaco tip.

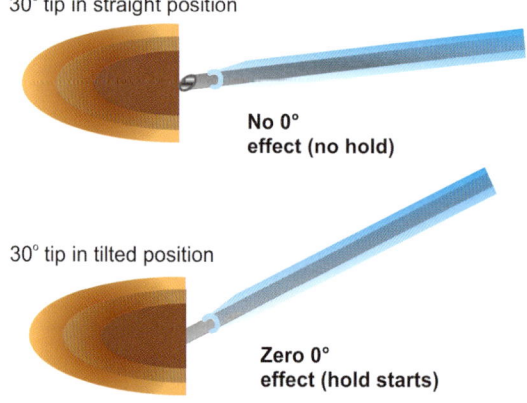

Fig. 3: Principles of hold.

■ PRINCIPLES OF HOLD (FIG. 3)

- In routine practice, 30° and 45° tips are used commonly. For a hold, one should place the phaco tip near the hard part of the nucleus to angle of the phaco tip in such a way that the phaco tip should give the 0° effect to the nuclear mass.
- Phaco tip should be engaged in the bulk of nucleus or the central hard part of the nuclear mass, with a minimal or an adequate energy to achieve the hold.
- To sustain or to maintain this hold, the 0° effect and engagement of the nucleus with minimal energy may be needed at frequent intervals.

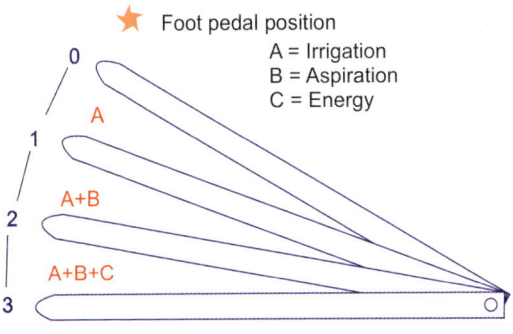

Fig. 4: Position of foot pedal.

ROLE OF VACUUM AND ASPIRATION FLOW RATES

- Aspiration flow rate keeps the better opposition of the nuclear mass toward the phaco tip.
- Vacuum plays a big role in holding the nucleus. Vacuum builds up to the preset level once the tip is occluded or engaged nicely with the nuclear bulk and it maintains the hold.

ROLE OF ENERGY

The energy is used first to engage the nucleus, and then to maintain the hold.

POSITIONS OF FOOT PEDAL (FIG. 4)

- Foot pedal position 1 is irrigation.
- Foot pedal position 2 is irrigation aspiration.
- Foot pedal position 3 is irrigation aspiration and phaco energy.

FUNCTIONS OF FOOT PEDALS

Position 1: It is irrigation which is helpful to maintain the anterior chamber and for better visualization by dispersing the soft materials of the lens.

Continuous irrigation can be maintained throughout the surgery by the machine itself, so the surgeon should concentrate on foot positions 2 and 3.

Position 2: It is used to hold the engaged nucleus and to maintain this hold.

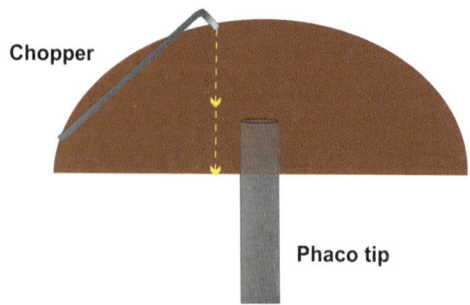
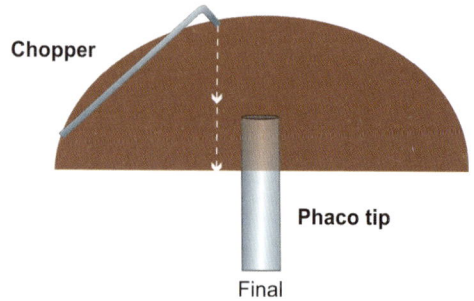

Fig. 5: Principles of chop.

Position 3: It is used to engage the nucleus.

Coordination of these foot positions from 3 to 2, 2 to 3, and repetition of these is one of the most important factors for hold of nucleus halve.

■ PRINCIPLES OF CHOP (FIG. 5)
- Chopping should be done only after holding the nucleus.
- *Chopping should always be in the bulk of the nucleus:* It means near to the phaco tip.
- Chopping should be done at 90° to the long axis of the nucleus, which means chopper should move parallel or near parallel to the phaco tip.

■ TYPES OF CHOPPING (FIGS. 6A AND B)
- *Horizontal chop:* When chopping is done at the round edge of the nucleus.

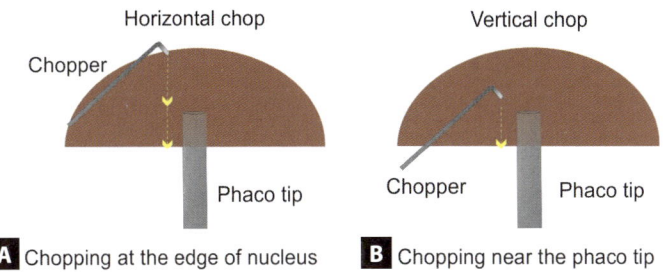

Figs. 6A and B: Types of chopping: (A) Horizontal and (B) Vertical.

TABLE 1: Parameters of hold and chop (phaco II).		
Energy	**Vacuum**	**Aspiration flow rate**
30–50% According to the density of nucleus	200–400 mm Hg	26–40 cc/min
Linear	Panel/Linear	Panel/Linear
Continuous		

- *Vertical chop:* When chopping is not possible from the round edge of the nucleus, then it is done near the phaco tip by moving the chopper in a vertical fashion in the mass of the nucleus, near the phaco tip till the posterior aspect of the nucleus and displace the pieces in opposite directions.

PARAMETER OF HOLD AND CHOP (PHACO II) (TABLE 1)

Following are commonly used parameters for hold. There are some variations in parameters from case to case and from machine to machine. Surgeons should customize their own parameters with practice.

Some Variations

They are according to different grades of nucleus. In hard-nucleus energy, vacuum and aspiration flow rates are on higher side and in soft cataract, all these parameters are on lower side.

Energy

- Sometimes, instead of using continuous energy, many machines have the option of hyperpulse mode. This mode can be used as a continuous hyperpulse mode (new definition by the author), where on time is more than off time.
- Sometimes, pulse energy or hyperpulse (off time is more than on time) can be used to hold the nucleus in a soft cataract.

Vacuum

- Vacuum should be increased from 200 to 400 mm Hg or may be more in hard cataract.
- Vacuum should be decreased from 150 to 100 mm Hg to hold soft cataract.

Aspiration Flow Rate

It can be increased with hard cataract and decreased with the soft cataract.

■ PREREQUISITE FOR HOLD AND CHOP

- Bulk of the nucleus
- Flat surface of each halve of nucleus
- Proper position of the nucleus is important for the hold. The surgeon should achieve the 0° effect with the respective nuclear mass in an easy way.
- Visualization of the working area should be better.
- Primary position of the eyeball—many times is needed.
- Complete division of the nucleus into two halves.

■ ROTATION OF NUCLEUS

- This is an important maneuver needed during this step of nucleus management.
- Rotation of nucleus is important for desire position for hold and chop.

■ PRINCIPLES OF ROTATION (FIGS. 7A AND B)

- Two instruments needed for two nucleus pieces **(Box 1)**
- One instrument is needed for one nucleus piece.

Hold and Chop of Nucleus

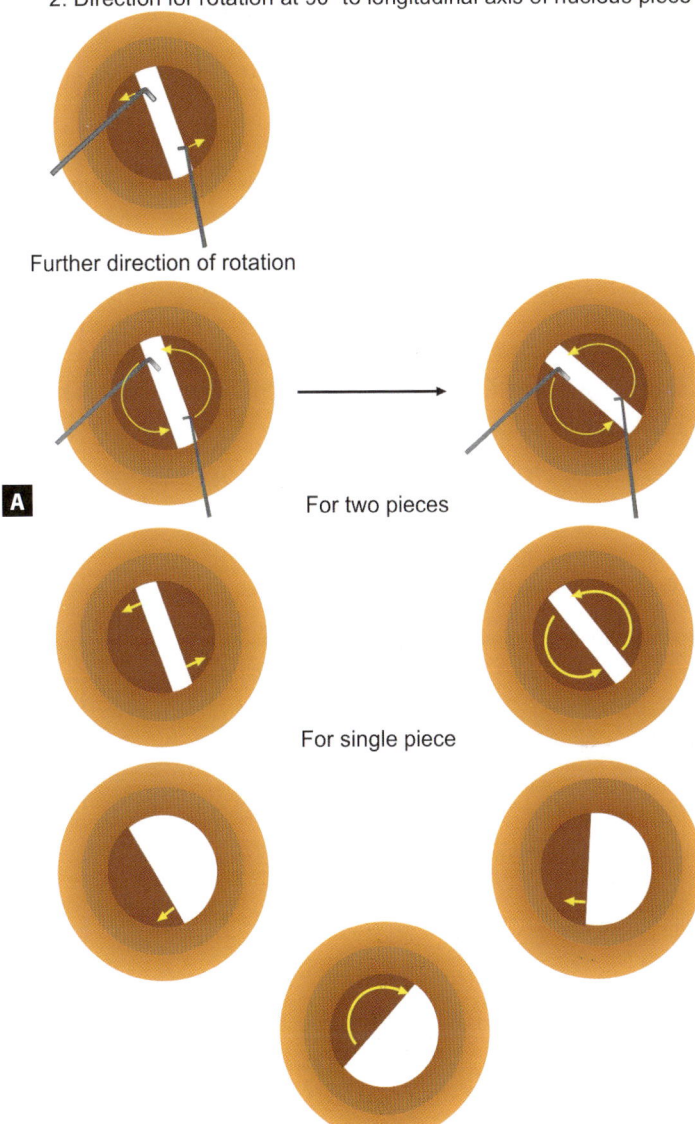

Figs. 7A and B: (A) Principles of rotation of nucleus and (B) Rotation of the nucleus to achieve the desire position of hold.

128 Hold and Chop of Nucleus

> **BOX 1:** Instruments needed for rotation of two nucleus pieces.
> - Dialer–dialer
> - Dialer–chopper
> - Viscocannula–chopper
> - Phaco tip–chopper

- Placement of instruments for rotation is near the periphery.
- Direction of movement or little force should be 90° to longitudinal axis of nucleus.
- Anterior chamber and bag should be well formed throughout the procedure.

CORRELATION OF HOLD AND CHOP WITH FOOT PEDAL (FIGS. 8A TO C)

Procedure of Hold and Horizontal Chop—Basic

- In a stop and chop technique after trench and division, one has to hold and chop each half of the nucleus.
- You can manage the right or the left hemisphere of the nucleus.

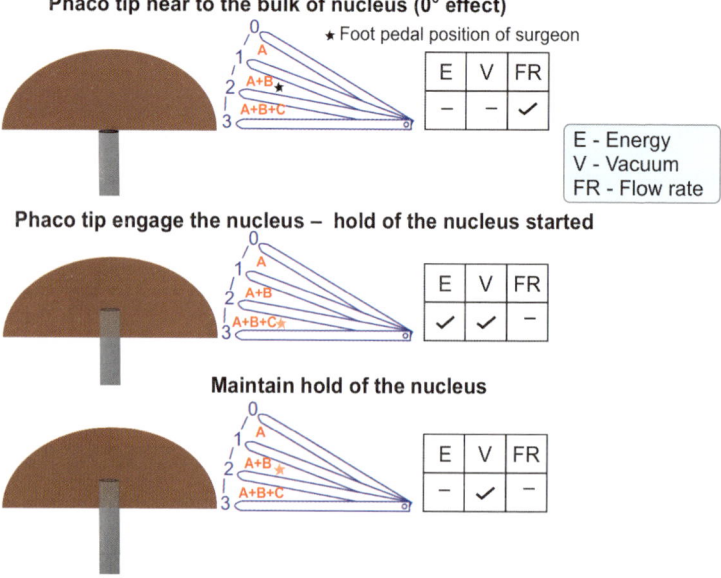

Fig. 8A

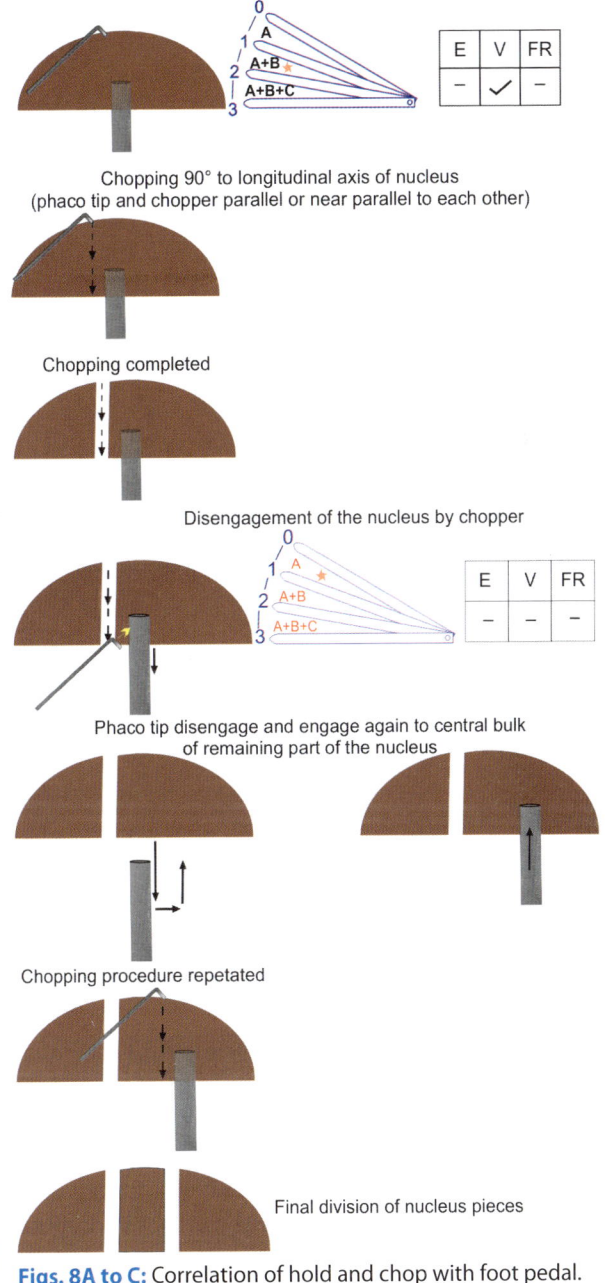

Figs. 8A to C: Correlation of hold and chop with foot pedal.

Hold and Chop of Nucleus

- When the two halves of nucleus are in situ, managing the first half of the nucleus is a real art in phaco surgery as working space is less.

Considering the Right Half of the Nucleus

The steps of hold and chop are as follows **(Figs. 9A and B)**:
1. Give the proper position to the right hemisphere of the nucleus.
2. Insert the phaco tip in the anterior chamber and place it near the right hemisphere in the groove of division and then start irrigation aspiration only which clears the soft material or debris which has been delivered during the trench.

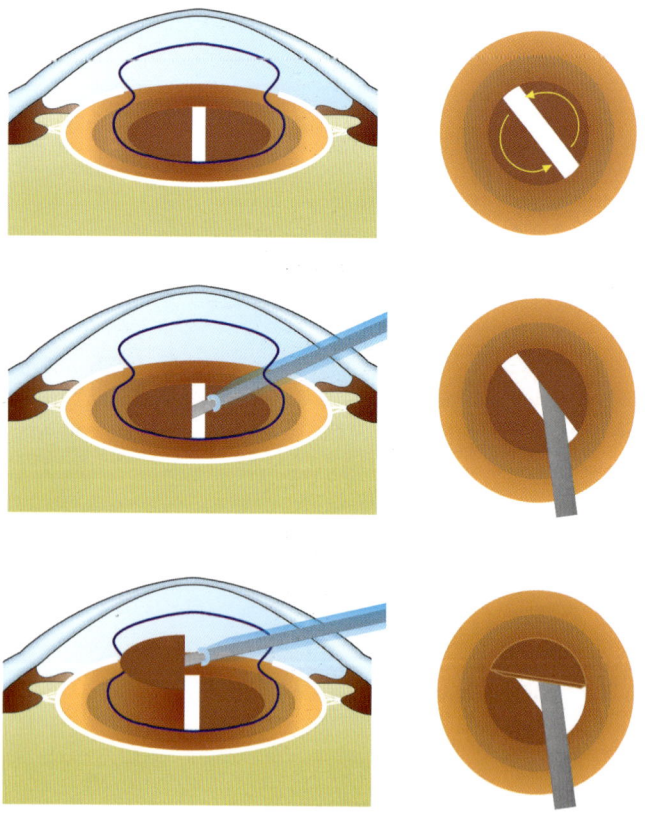

Fig. 9A

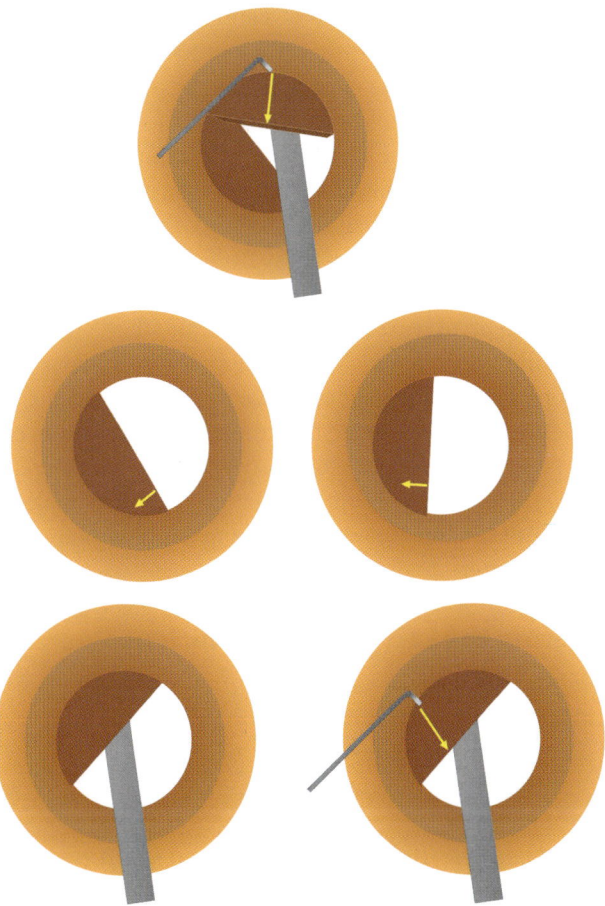

Fig. 9B

Figs. 9A and B: Procedure of hold and chop.

3. Phaco tip should be placed at the center and hold the nucleus. This holding of the nucleus has to be maintained by foot pedal position 2. Now, lift the inferior edge of the nucleus out of the bag; to achieve this, phaco tip should move superiorly, then lift the piece using your wrist movement and do all manipulations (principles of hold) with aiming to bring inferior edge of the nucleus out of the bag and chop it.

4. Phaco tip should be placed at center of the right hemisphere of the nucleus, keeping the 0° effect at the central mass; use minimum or adequate energy to engage the nucleus. Once the nucleus is engaged, hold starts. According to the author, the most important step is one should learn to maintain the hold for a longer time. Without losing the hold on the nucleus, it is lifted out of the bag very slowly. Usually, lift the inferior edge first and chop it. Then release the nucleus away from the phaco tip by chopper and reengage the remaining part of nucleus in central position by moving the phaco tip toward right side and then chop again.
5. One of the important factors for chopping of nucleus is that the position of the nucleus should be central and horizontal; it means parallel or near to parallel to the iris plain and away from cornea so that placement of chopper to pass over the nucleus for reaching at the edge of nucleus is easy and chopping becomes simple and safe.
6. Removal of small pieces after chopping will be explained in detail in next chapter.

Considering the Left Half of the Nucleus

Following are the steps for hold and chop:
1. This is relatively easy as there is more space.
2. Rotate the nucleus in desired position.
3. Repeat the same procedure.
4. *Some differences:*
    a. To keep the nucleus in horizontal position, phaco tip should be moved in clockwise direction after hold for better chopping.
    b. Chopping the left side of nucleus has a restricted movement of chopper as distance between chopper and nucleus is less.

■ VARIATIONS FOR HOLD (FIG. 10)

Bulk of nucleus is better for hold. Elevated mass is better for hold.

■ VERTICAL CHOP

- When surgeon cannot reach the edge of nucleus to chop (horizontal chop), he has to consider vertical chop.

Hold and Chop of Nucleus

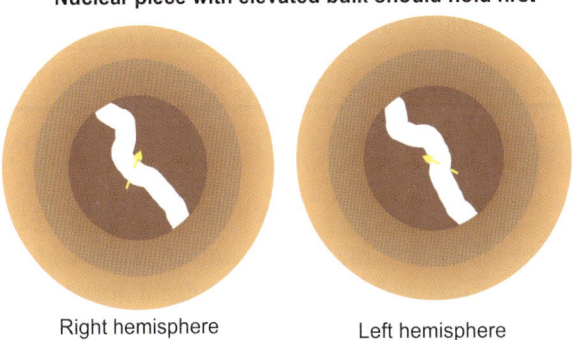

Fig. 10: Variations for hold.

- *Indications:*
  - Very hard cataract
  - Small capsulorhexis
  - Cataract with big-size nucleus
  - Cataract with hazy cornea
  - Cataract with shallow anterior chamber
  - Cataract with small pupil

■ COMPLICATIONS DURING HOLD AND CHOP

Following complications are observed during hold and chop:
- Anterior capsule tear
- Corneal injury due to chopper
- Posterior capsular rent
- *Zonular dialysis:* Due to more pressure of chopper on nucleus
- Posterior subluxation or dislocation of the lens
- Trauma to the iris
- Surge

■ DIFFICULTIES DURING HOLD AND CHOP

Following difficulties are observed during hold and chop:
- Inadequate hold
- More or less energy used during chopping
- Chopping without hold

- Hold at periphery
- Lifting of nucleus with fast movement

DIFFICULT SITUATIONS FOR HOLD AND CHOP

Following are the difficult situations for hold and chop:
- Soft cataract
- Very hard cataract
- Sticky cataract

ROLE OF CHOPPER

Following are the roles of chopper:
- For division of nucleus
- Chopping of the nucleus
- Release the piece of nucleus away from the phaco tip to rehold it in a better position and chop.
- Release the pieces of nucleus to reorient them for easy emulsifying of small piece.
- Sometimes, for rotation of nucleus
- To stabilize the globe that facilitates all steps of phaco surgery in topical anesthesia
- To give the proper position of eyeball in topical anesthesia
- To push the pieces of nucleus back into the anterior chamber which are stuck at the side port
- During irrigation aspiration, to feed the sticky epinucleus by clearing the aspiration port of irrigation aspiration canula

MISUSE OF CHOPPER

- To bring the nucleus pieces toward the phaco tip, which has been routinely practiced, but the author thinks that aspiration flow rate is responsible for bringing the nucleus pieces toward phaco tip and chopper is to reorient them. This is called feeding the nucleus by releasing it. This is inverse or reverse feeding.
- Removal of pieces of nucleus by hitting the chopper to the phaco tip.

Hold and Chop of Nucleus

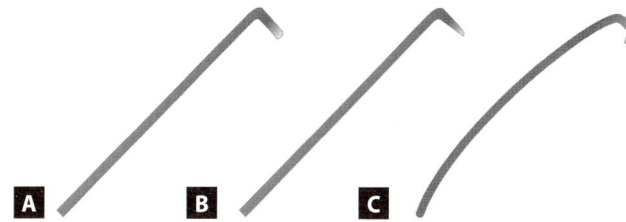

Figs. 11A to C: Types of choppers: (A) Nagahara chopper; (B) Sharp chopper; and (C) Toshniwal chopper.

■ PLACEMENT OF CHOPPER

- Chopper should go in horizontally and should come out horizontally.
- During the chopping, it is placed vertically, i.e., at 90° or near 90° to the long axis of nucleus.
- During the removal of small pieces, to reorient the nucleus pieces, chopper should be placed horizontally, i.e., parallel to iris.
- Keep the chopper near to the side port incision of entry horizontally when it is not working. This is called resting position of chopper.

■ TYPES OF CHOPPERS (FIGS. 11A TO C)

- *Nagahara chopper:* This basic chopper has cutting edge and blunt tip.
- *Sharp chopper with pointed tip:* May be for hard cataract
- *Toshniwal chopper:* Modification of Nagahara chopper with curved shaft and length of distal end is lesser.

■ COMPLICATIONS DUE TO THE CHOPPER

Following complications occurred due to the chopper:
- Descemet's membrane detachment
- Iris trauma
- Anterior capsule tear
- Posterior capsular rent
- Endothelial damage
- Epithelial damage

- More pressure at the incision site:
  - Shallow anterior chamber
  - Iris prolapse from side port
  - Surge
- Damage to the phaco tip and sleeve

SPEED OF THE CHOPPER

In most of the steps concerned with the chopper, the movement of chopper should be very slow.

KEY POINTS

- Ideal trench and division are the most important prerequisite for hold and chop.
- 0° effect—bulk of the nucleus is essential for hold.
- Foot pedal positions, especially from two to three and back, are to be practiced to maintain the hold.
- Chopping should be always at 90° to the long axis of nucleus piece and in the bulk—means chopper moves parallel or near to parallel to phaco tip.
- Ideal hold and chop will assist in removal of small pieces.
- In this step of hold and chop, hold is more important as the surgeon cannot chop ideally without a proper hold.

LIVE SURGERY PHOTOGRAPHS

For One Half of Nucleus (Figs. 12A to N)

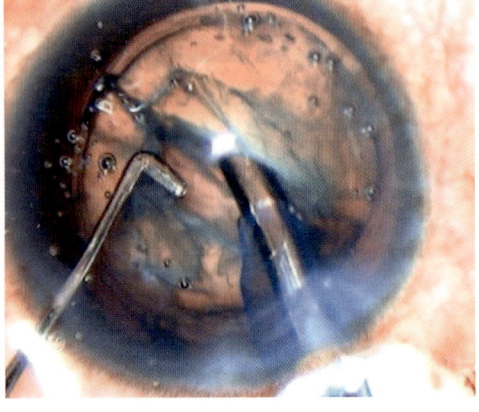

Fig. 12A: Hold and chop. A perfect 0° effect at the central hard part of nucleus (chopper placed horizontally).

Hold and Chop of Nucleus

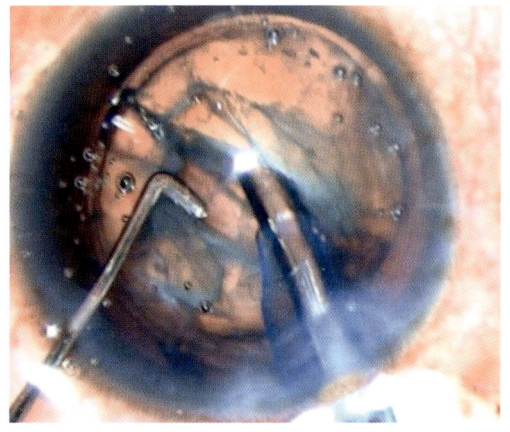

Fig. 12B: Foot pedal position 2 to remove the soft tissue for better visualization and started better apposition.

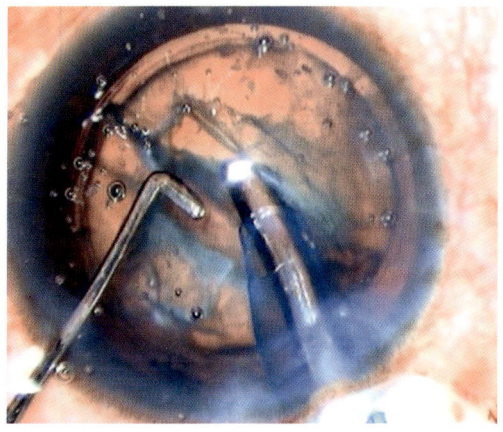

Fig. 12C: Engage the phaco tip with adequate energy (foot pedal position 3). This starts hold of nucleus.

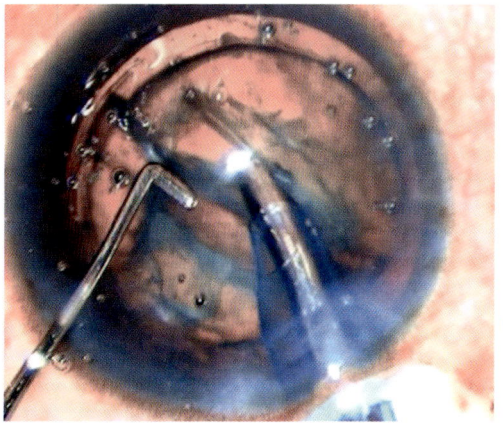

Fig. 12D: Maintain the hold and start lifting the nucleus half in foot pedal position 2.

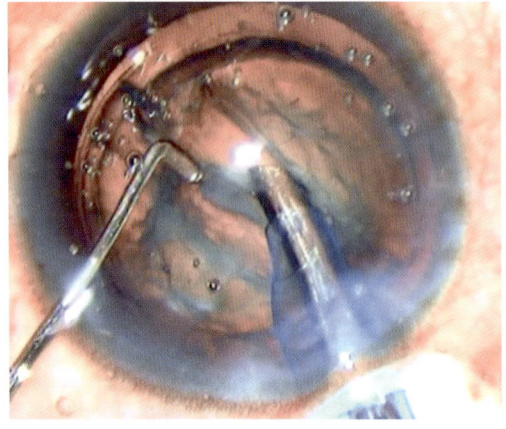

Fig. 12E: Nucleus has separated from its epinucleus which indicates better hold in foot pedal position 2.

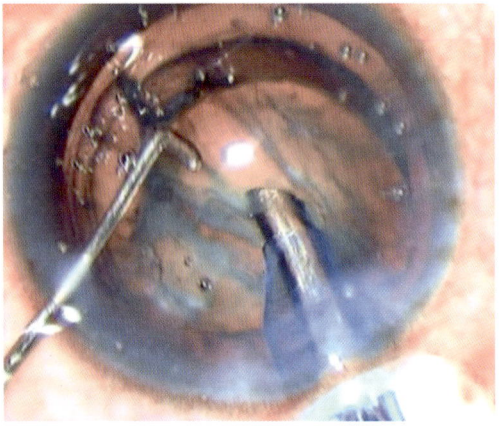

Fig. 12F: Bring the inferior nucleus edge at the level of capsulorhexis. Foot pedal position 2.

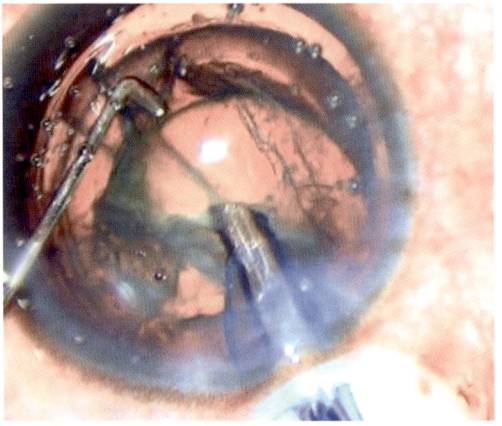

Fig. 12G: Tilted nucleus halve in CSZ near capsulorhexis plane, ready for chop with placement of chopper at the edge of nucleus. Foot pedal position 2.

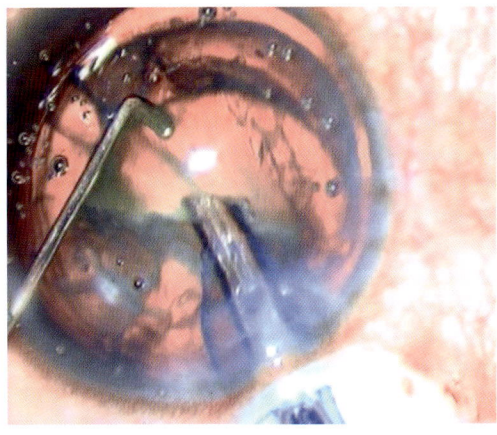

Fig. 12H: Direction of chopping, 90° to the longitudinal axis of the nucleus halve, means parallel to phaco tip.

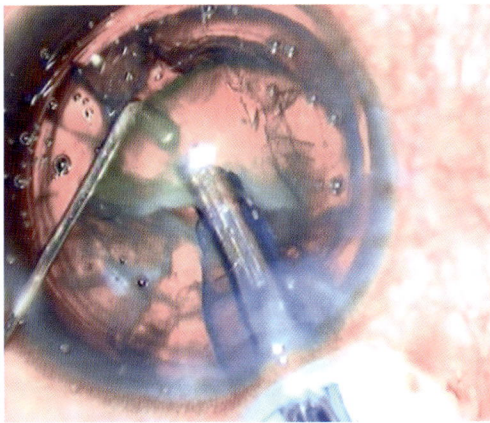

Fig. 12I: Direction of force toward the phaco tip. Foot pedal position 2.

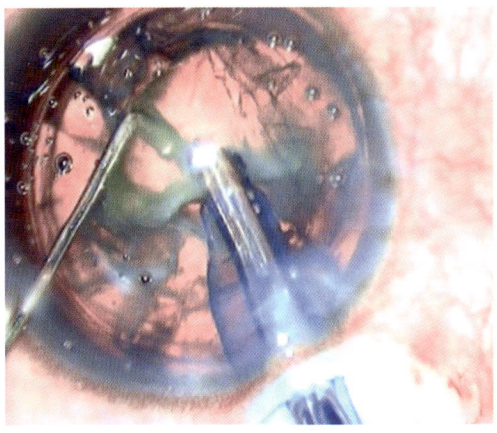

Fig. 12J: Horizontal chopping.

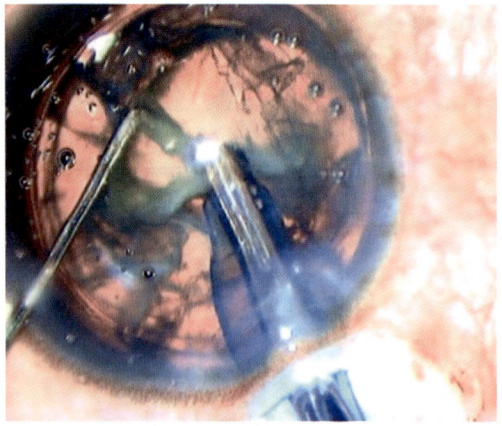

Fig. 12K: Chopping completed.

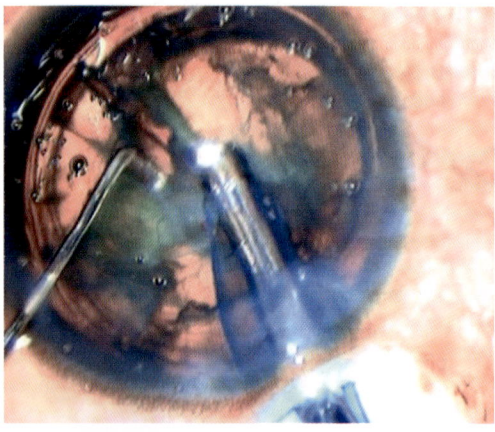

Fig. 12L: Piece displaced away from main piece.

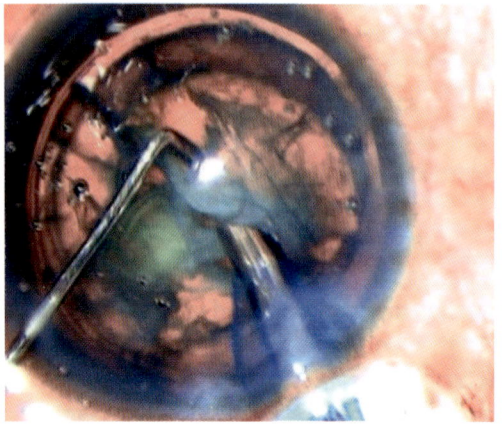

Fig. 12M: Rehold the remaining nucleus piece in the center.

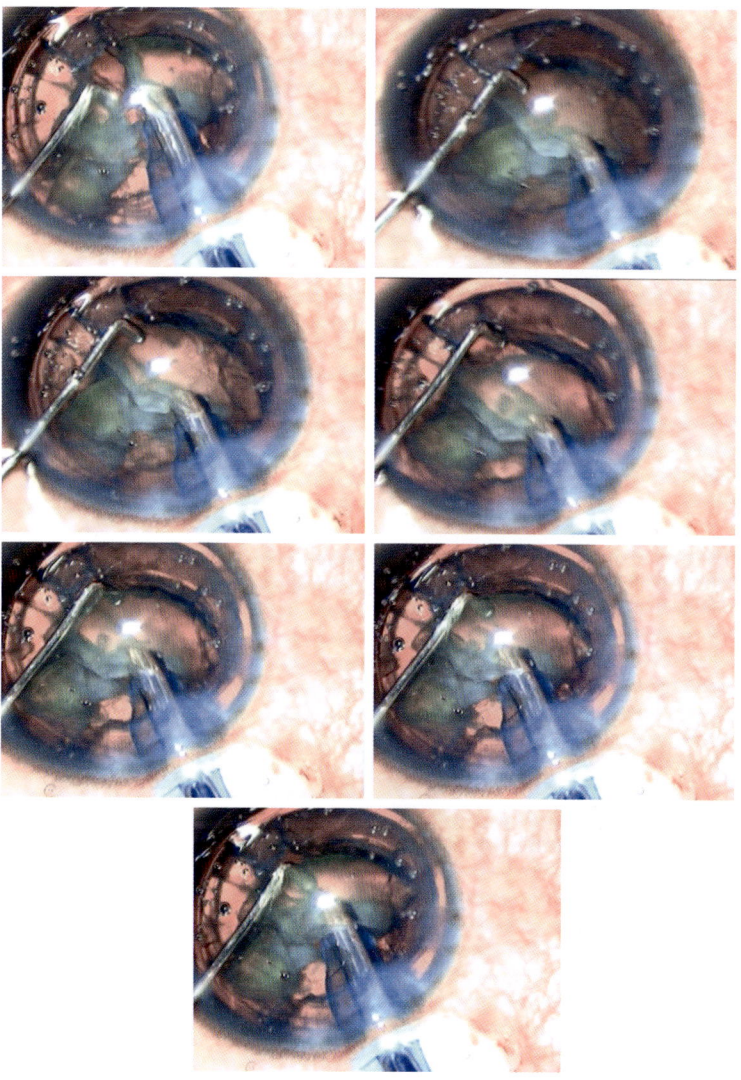

Fig. 12N: Procedure is repeated.

Hold and Chop of Nucleus

For Other Side of Nucleus (Figs. 13A to I)

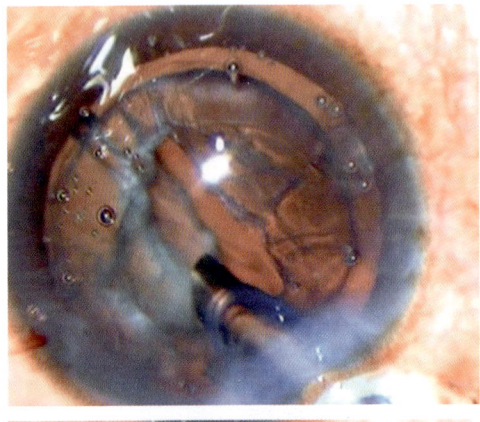

Fig. 13A: For removal of left half of nucleus, phaco tip reoriented. Foot pedal position 2.

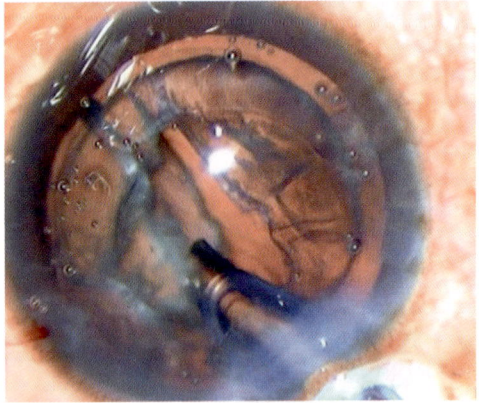

Fig. 13B: 0° effect in the central bulk of the nucleus.

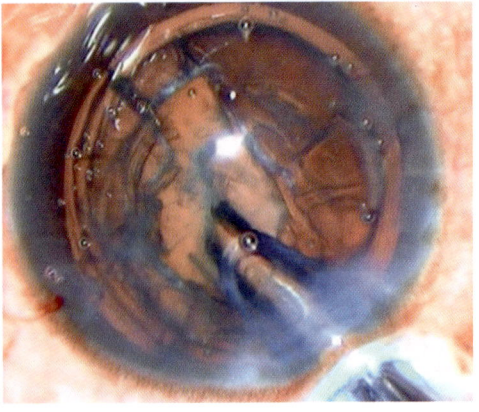

Fig. 13C: Engage the nucleus with adequate energy and lift. Foot pedal position 3.

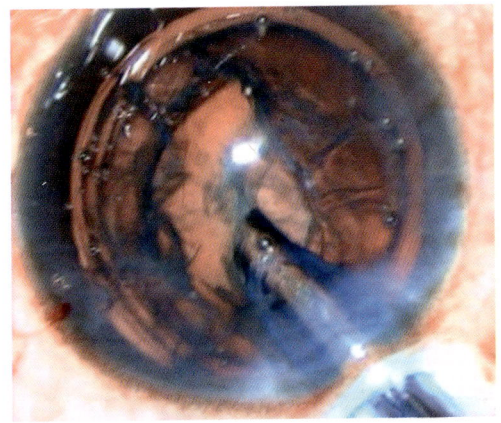

Fig. 13D: Lifting of second half of nucleus is easy as there is more space.

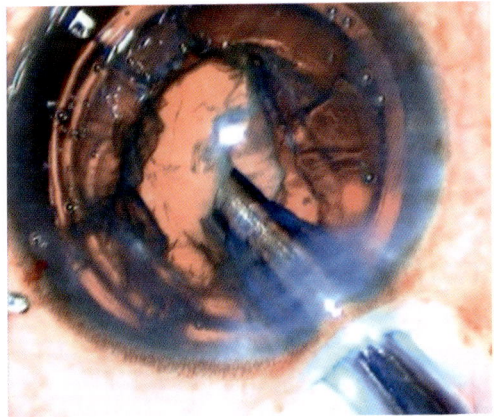

Fig. 13E: Reorient the nucleus mass from tilted position to horizontal position for easy and safe chopping.

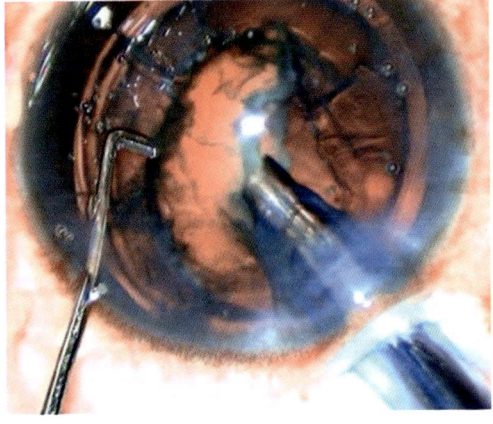

Fig. 13F: Phaco tip and chopper placed at perfect position for horizontal chopping.

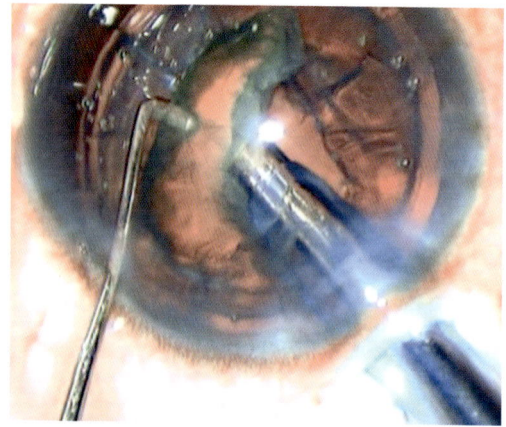

Fig. 13G: In foot pedal position 2, chopping started.

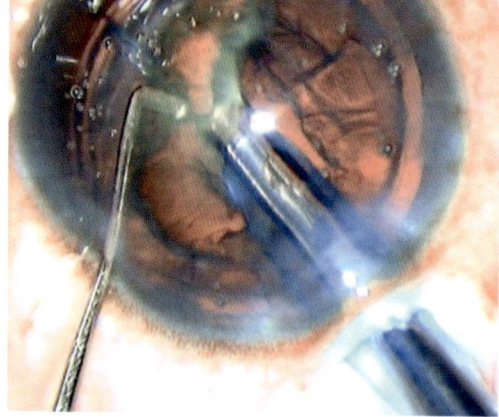

Fig. 13H: Direction of chopper toward the phaco tip.

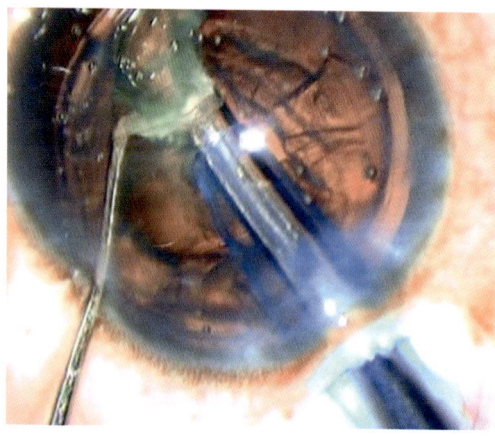

Fig. 13I: Chopping completed.

CHAPTER 12

Removal of Small Pieces of Nucleus

■ INTRODUCTION

Although this is a simple step in nucleus management, complications such as posterior capsule rupture (PCR), injury to anterior capsule, iris trauma, and postoperative hazy cornea are common. So, to avoid this, surgeons should know specific area or safe zone to remove small pieces. One should know specific parameters and factors or instruments which are having the real role in removal of nucleus pieces.

■ INSTRUMENTS (FIG. 1)

Following are the instruments used in removal of small pieces:
- Chopper
- Phaco tip
- Viscoelastic and viscocannula

■ PRINCIPLE

Aspiration flow rate: It is one of the most important parameters to bring the nuclear pieces toward phaco tip.

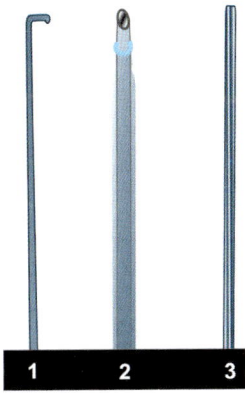

Fig. 1: Instruments: (1) Chopper; (2) Phaco tip; (3) Viscocannula.

146 Removal of Small Pieces of Nucleus

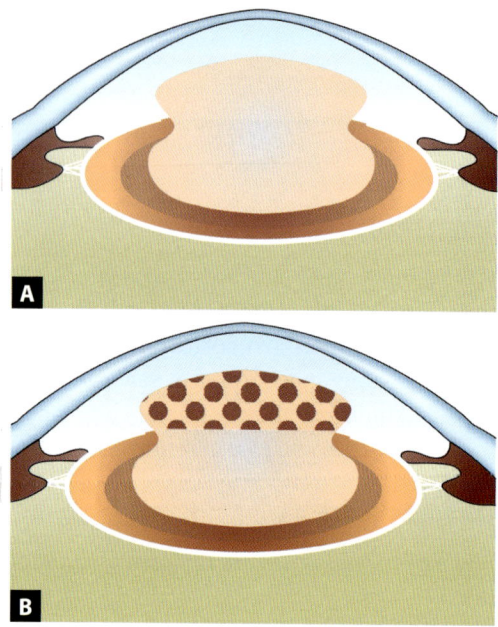

Figs. 2A and B: Ideal site to remove small pieces: (A) Safe zone for phaco surgery—central safe zone (CSZ) and (B) Safe zone to remove small pieces of nucleus.

Energy: Once the piece is in opposition, use minimum energy to engage the nucleus or sometimes, use energy to bring the nucleus in opposition and engage. Energy is used to emulsify the nuclear pieces.

Vacuum: It builds up once nucleus is engaged. Then start using adequate or minimum energy for emulsifying the pieces.

■ IDEAL SITE TO REMOVE SMALL PIECES (FIGS. 2A AND B)

In **Figures 2A and B**, safe zone for phaco surgery is demarcated. Part which is out of bag of that area (posterior aspect of anterior chamber) is most ideal and safe site to remove small pieces.

■ PARAMETERS (TABLE 1—PHACO III)

See **Table 1**.

Removal of Small Pieces of Nucleus

TABLE 1: Parameters for removal of small pieces.

Energy	Vacuum	Aspiration flow rate
20–40% According to the density of nucleus	200–300 mm Hg	24–30 cc/min
Traditional pulse or hyperpulse	Linear or panel	Linear or panel

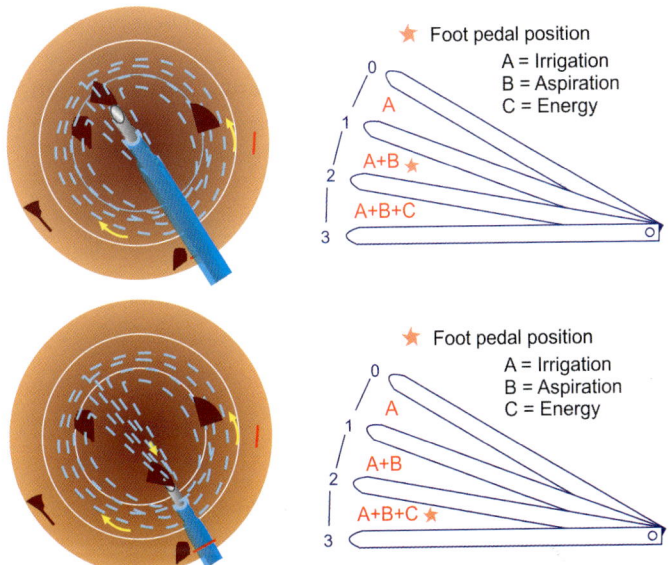

Fig. 3: Correlation of foot pedal with parameter.

CORRELATION OF FOOT PEDAL WITH PARAMETER—MOST IMPORTANT (FIG. 3)

Foot pedal positions 2 and 3 play a significant role in this step.

Foot pedal position 2 brings the piece toward tip and then foot pedal position 3 emulsifies it.

ROLE OF ENERGY, VACUUM, AND FLOW RATE

Energy
- Pulse or hyperpulse
- Minimum or adequate, i.e., 20–40%
- To engage the piece

- Once engaged, to emulsify the pieces
- Energy should be used according to the different zones of nucleus; hard part of nucleus needs relatively more energy, and soft part needs relatively less energy.
- Energy used in the central zone can be more, but it should be less than adequate as tip is moving toward periphery and toward cornea or posterior capsule.
- Sometimes, energy is needed to hold and chop nucleus pieces during removal of small pieces.
- Sometimes when epinucleus is coming along with nucleus, energy may be needed to remove epinucleus also.
- Energy should be cut down for last pieces removal.

Modes of Energy (Figs. 4A and B)
- Traditional pulse mode
- *Hyperpulse mode:* May be in the form of continuous hyperpulse or pulse hyperpulse (new definition by author)
- *How these parameters work:*
  - Energy cuts
  - Gap holds
- *Pulse energy:* Cut-hold-cut-hold
  - So that pulse mode is more controlled and safer
- Setting is four to six pulses per second

Energy Used in Wrong Way
Some illustrations are as follows (Figs. 5A and B):
- Energy used is more than needed, so repulsion of piece is called chatter.
- Energy used in empty space, so cornea gets hazy

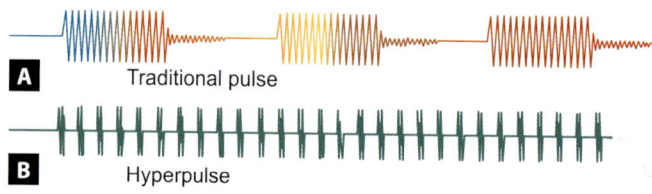

Figs. 4A and B: Modes of energy: (A) Traditional pulse and (B) Hyperpulse.

Removal of Small Pieces of Nucleus

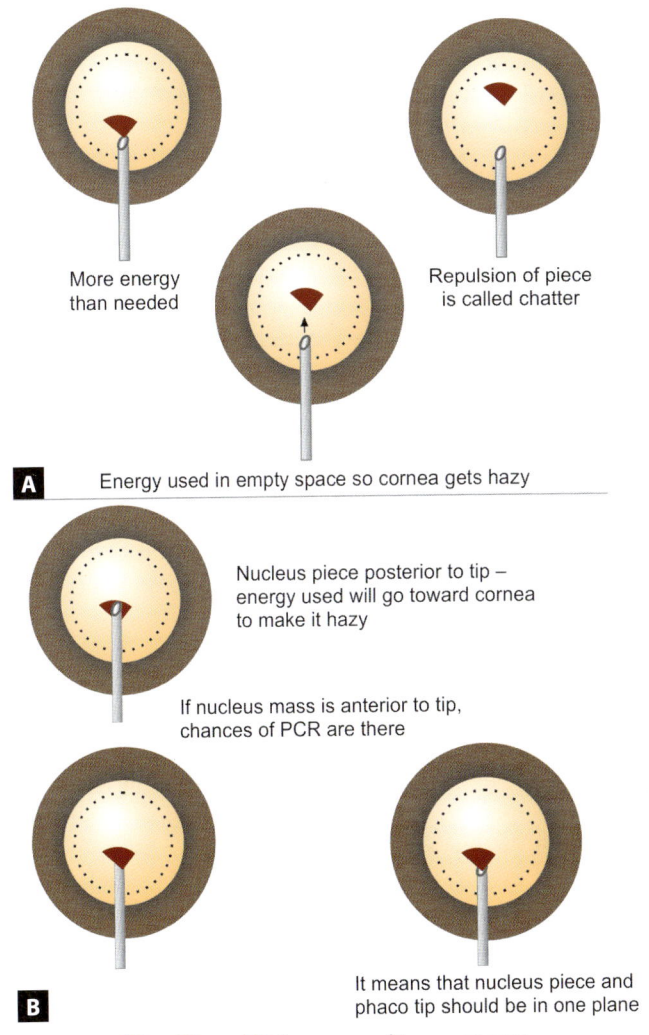

Figs. 5A and B: Energy used in wrong way.

- Energy used in the vicinity of nucleus piece but without engaging to it, which is also responsible for postoperative hazy cornea
- *Nucleus piece posterior to tip:* Energy used will go toward cornea to make it hazy.
- If nucleus mass is anterior to tip, chances of PCR are there.

It means that nucleus piece and phaco tip should be in one plane.

Vacuum

- Once nucleus engaged, vacuum builds up to keep the piece in engaged position or to keep the piece in opposition of tip—this is nothing but hold. Emulsification of nucleus after this hold will make procedure more effective and very safe.
- Adequate vacuum is needed for this procedure.
- It ranges from 150 to 300 mm Hg for routine cases and should be more, i.e., 300–400 mm Hg in hard cataract.
- It can be in linear or panel mode.
- Vacuum is to hold; maintain the hold before use of energy.
- Sometimes with vacuum, surgeon can emulsify soft nucleus.

Vacuum used in wrong way: Misconception about vacuum is that when pieces are not coming toward the phaco tip, surgeons are increasing the vacuum which has no specific role for that purpose.

If a surgeon fails to remove pieces, then out of frustration surgeon increases vacuum.

Aspiration Flow Rate

- Understanding of phaco fluidics in this step means understanding of flow rate which plays a vital role in emulsification of small pieces.
- By definition, flow rate means the followability of the tissue, which means pieces which are moving toward the phaco tip are due to flow rate.
- It should be adequate, i.e., 24–30 cc/min.
- It should be usually linear; panel can be used for faster work.

Factors which are assisting the flow rate:
- Horizontal position of globe
- Water current of irrigation fluid
- If phaco tip is in bevel-up or near to bevel-up, water currents move in horizontal fashion to facilitate bringing nucleus pieces toward tip.
- More number of leakages or more number of instruments decreases flow rate.

Some facts related to flow rate: Depends on water current **(Figs. 6A and B)**, if two instruments phaco tip and chopper (through two openings) are placed in anterior chamber, water current diverts due to leakage, so flow rate decreases.

If only one instrument, phaco tip (through one opening), is placed in the anterior chamber, there is no leakage, so effectivity of flow rate is nearly equal to preset parameter (near to 100%).

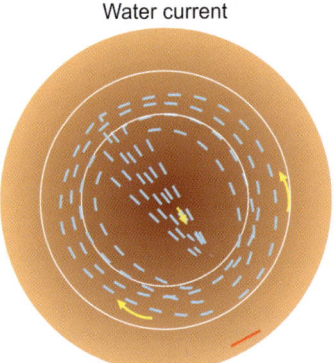

Correlation of flow rate with number of openings and instruments in the anterior chamber

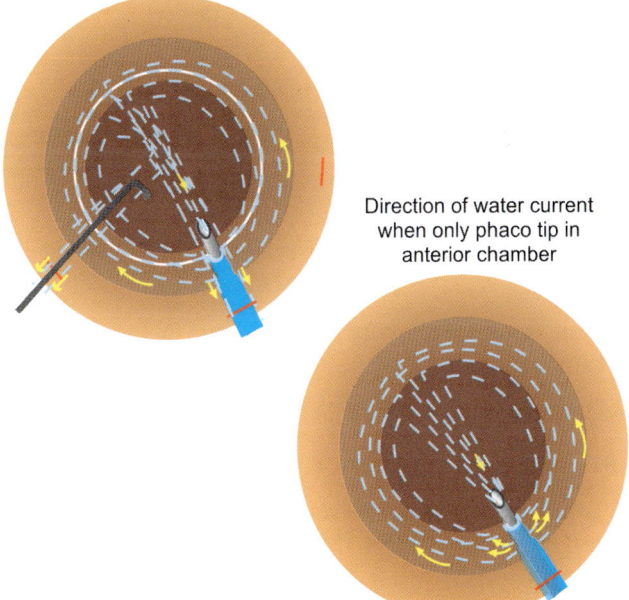

Fig. 6A

Removal of Small Pieces of Nucleus

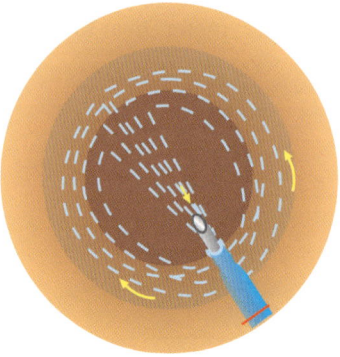

Direction of water current when only phaco tip in anterior chamber

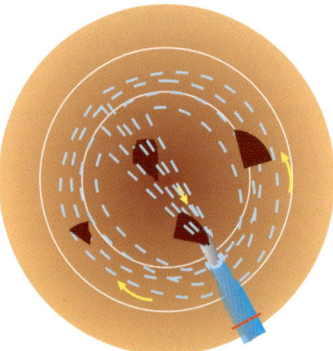

Direction of the small nuclear pieces Directed toward phaco tip (aspiration flow rate working at its preset parameter 100% or near to it)

Fig. 6B

Figs. 6A and B: Water current.

Sometimes, surgeons increase flow rate for fast removal of pieces, but caution should be taken as chances of catching of iris and PCR increases.

■ PHACO TIP

- *Placement of phaco tip inside the chamber* **(Figs. 7A and B)**:
  - Placement of phaco tip should be in central safe zone, i.e., in the center or just behind it.
  - Phaco tip moves toward the periphery to engage nucleus piece and brings toward center for further emulsification.

Removal of Small Pieces of Nucleus

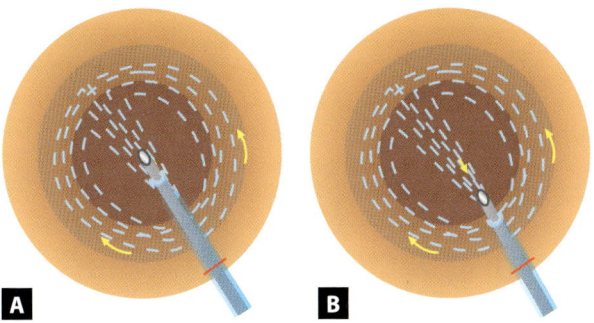

Figs. 7A and B: Ideal placement of phaco tip during removal of small pieces: (A) Placement of phaco tip should be in the center and (B) Just behind the center.

During this maneuver, press the foot pedal partially to decrease the parameter.
- Phaco tip should be in bevel-up or bevel lateral position during emulsification of nuclear pieces.
- Direction of phaco tip may be bevel-up, sideway, or down to give 0° effect to engage nucleus.

■ *Movement of phaco tip during this step should be very slow for following reasons:*
  - Complication rate decreases
  - There is no turbulence of water current
  - Correlation of foot pedal with phaco tip is better.

Orientation of nucleus pieces with phaco tip is most crucial factor for effective and safe procedure **(Figs. 8A to E)**.
- Try to catch the long axis of pieces for larger working distance for better efficiency of energy and it is always safe.
- Try to get the apex of the piece.
- Try to catch the edge of nucleus piece.
- Try to catch the bulk of nucleus.
- Avoid catching from round surface of nucleus piece.

■ ROLE OF CHOPPER (FIGS. 9A AND B)
- Placement of chopper should be in horizontal position.
- For easy maneuvering of position of eyeball or fixation of eyeball
- To chop the big nucleus pieces and partial chopping or teasing of nucleus

Removal of Small Pieces of Nucleus

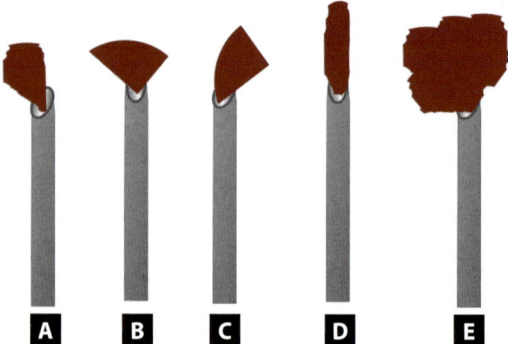

Figs. 8A to E: Orientation of nucleus pieces with phaco tip: (A and B) Catch at apex of nucleus piece; (C) Catch at the edge and apex of nucleus piece; (D) Catch at the long axis of nucleus piece; and (E) Catch the bulk of nucleus mass.

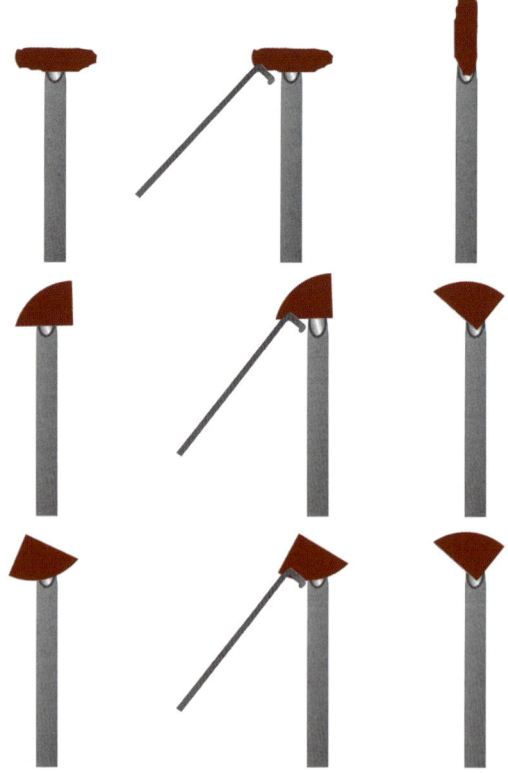

Fig. 9A

Removal of Small Pieces of Nucleus

Try to keep the pieces in horizontal position, which is parallel to iris

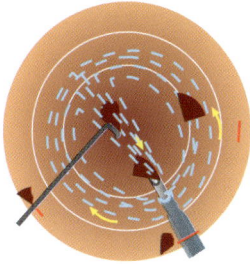 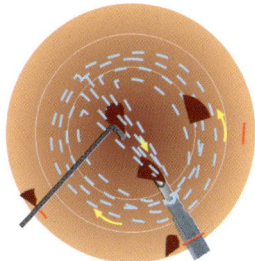

Try to keep the piece away from cornea

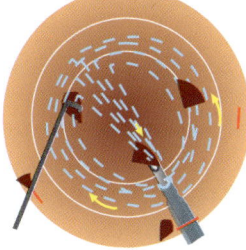

Push the nucleus piece from incision site at the same time phaco tip is in catching position

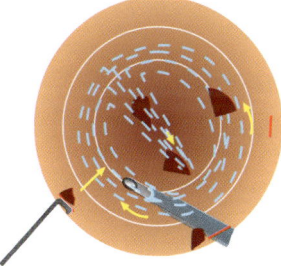

Fig. 9B

Figs. 9A and B: (A) Role of chopper for reorientation of nucleus pieces and (B) Role of chopper in removal of small pieces.

- Reorientation or guiding of nucleus pieces toward phaco tip by disengaging the nucleus or by pushing nucleus piece away from phaco tip
- Keep horizontal plane of nucleus pieces which are wandering in the anterior chamber.

Removal of Small Pieces of Nucleus

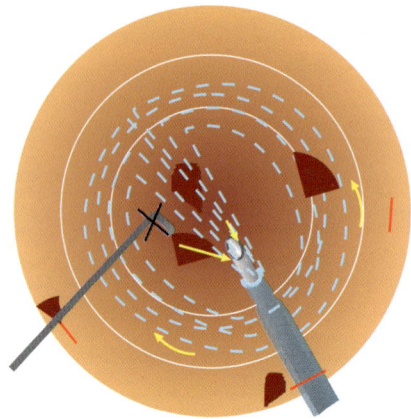

Use of chopper for bringing the pieces towards phaco tip

Fig. 10: Misuse of chopper.

- To keep or maintain same plane of phaco tip and nucleus piece
- Try to keep nucleus pieces away from cornea.
- To push the pieces of nucleus which got stuck at side port incision
- Minimum use of chopper for removal of small pieces is more effective.

■ MISUSE OF CHOPPER (FIG. 10)

To bring nucleus pieces toward phaco tip.

Disadvantage of Chopper

Water current diverts toward side port, so effectivity of flow rate decreases.

■ VISCOELASTICS AND VISCOCANNULA

- To inflate the anterior chamber and bag
- Keep the pieces away from cornea and posterior capsule.
- Try to bring the pieces toward the safe zone.
- Try to push the pieces in the center, which get stuck at incision sites.
- If tubings get blocked by nucleus pieces and phaco stops working—at this movement, phaco tip should move out of

Removal of Small Pieces of Nucleus

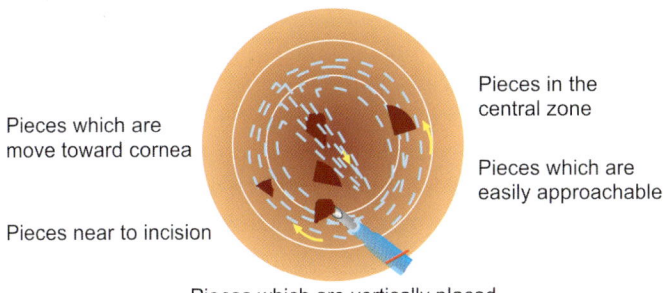

Fig. 11: Which piece to remove first.

anterior chamber and it should be inflated by putting viscoelastics through side port.
- Small pieces of nucleus can be removed by viscoelastics.

Which Pieces to Remove First (Fig. 11)
- This is not in the surgeon's hand as nucleus pieces are wandering here and there due to water current. Still, some points concerned with this will be helpful for this procedure.
- Nucleus pieces in central safe zone can be removed easily.
- Piece which moves toward cornea
- Pieces which are easily approachable to phaco tip
- If two pieces are there, the piece which is near to main incision should be removed first.
- If hard part of particular nucleus piece touching endothelium
- Big piece wandering in the anterior chamber should be tackled first.

Which Piece to Remove Last
- Nucleus piece which is near to posterior capsule
- Piece wandering in the bag
- Pieces which are awkwardly approachable to phaco tip.

■ COMPLICATIONS
As in other steps, these steps are also having some complications. Two most important complications are as follows:

Removal of Small Pieces of Nucleus

1. *Hazy cornea:*
   - Mechanical touching of phaco tip, chopper, viscocannula, and nucleus pieces
   - Sudden collapse of chamber due to surge during procedure
   - If nucleus pieces stay longer near cornea
   - If phaco tip is over the nucleus piece during removal
   - If preexisting shallow anterior chamber
   - Unnecessary use of energy in empty space of anterior chamber
   - Use of energy without opposition of nucleus or without engaging the nucleus
   - Use of energy near cornea
   - Sudden removal of phaco tip out of eye due to any reason collapses anterior chamber and nucleus pieces can hit the cornea.
2. *Posterior capsule rupture:*
   - Mechanical injury by phaco tip, chopper, and viscocannula
   - Use of wrong parameters near posterior capsule
   - Use of parameters without engaging nucleus pieces
   - Wrong placement of phaco tip with respect to nucleus pieces
   - Emulsification of pieces in the bag

■ KEY POINTS

Chances of PCR are very common in this step, so to understand all principles related to phaco fluidics and associated factors is mandatory.

■ LIVE SURGERY PHOTOGRAPHS (FIGS. 12A TO Z)

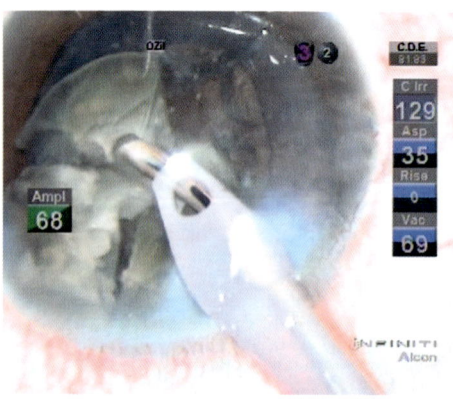

Fig. 12A: In torsional technology with Kelman tip, horizontal placement of tip, parallel to the nucleus mass is important for the removal of small pieces.

Removal of Small Pieces of Nucleus

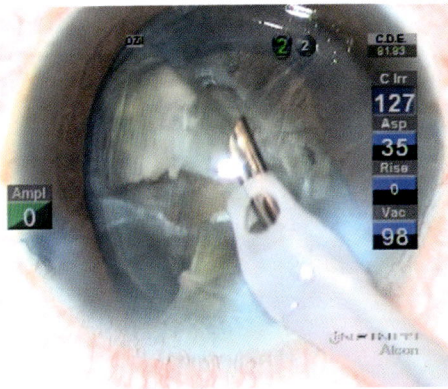

Fig. 12B: Bevel sideways to catch the apex of the nuclear mass.

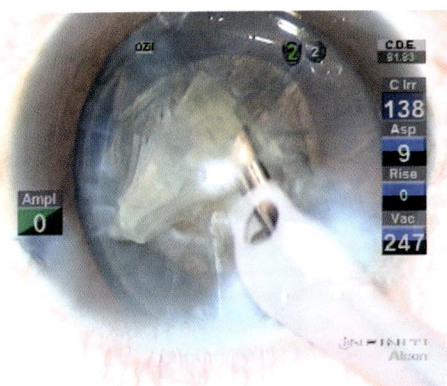

Fig. 12C: Placement of the phaco tip to round edge of the nucleus mass helps in speedy removal of nucleus mass which is opposite to longitudinal phaco.

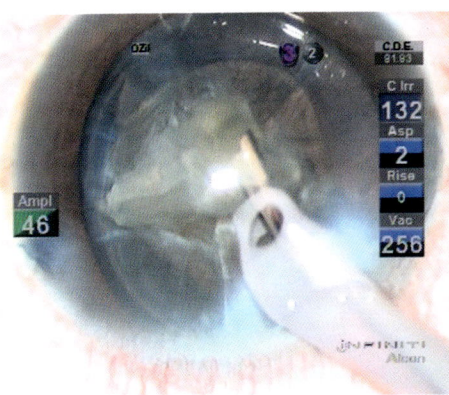

Fig. 12D: Torsional phaco energy started with adequate vacuum.

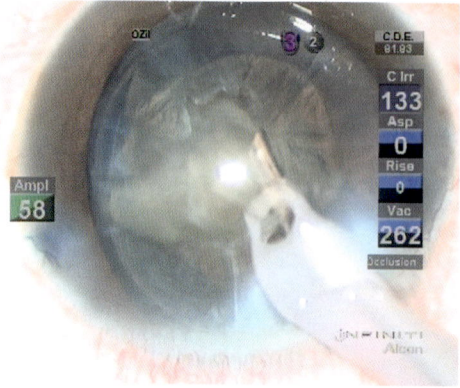

Fig. 12E: Nucleus is removed at the level of capsulorhexis or just anterior to it.

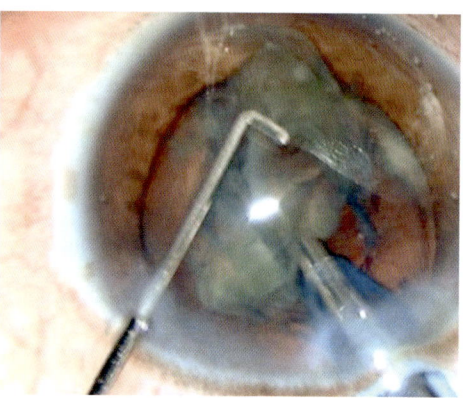

Fig. 12F: For hard nuclear mass, chopper assisting for chopping, teasing (partial chopping), reverse chopping, or release the piece for proper reorientation of nucleus mass for better emulsification.

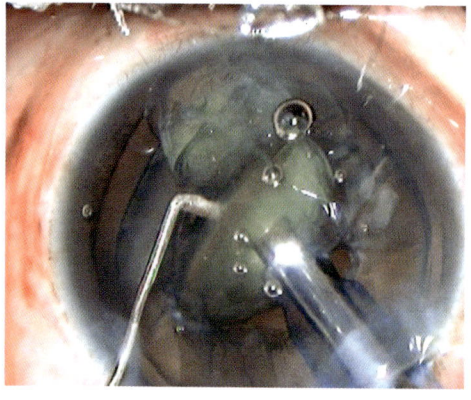

Fig. 12G: During emulsification, if bulk is big, chop first and then emulsify the piece.

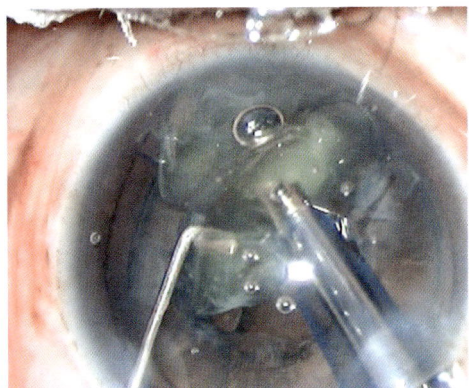

Fig. 12H: Chopping of the big piece is done.

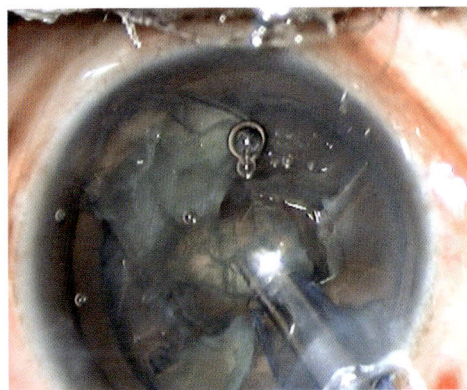

Fig. 12I: Emulsification of piece usually at the central safe zone (CSZ).

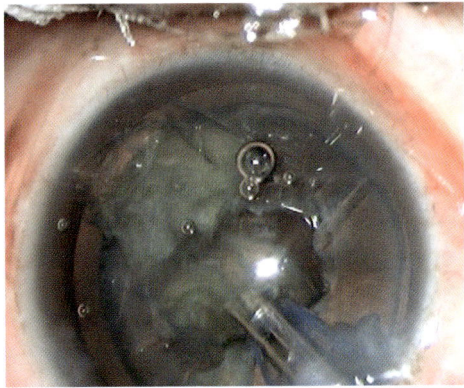

Fig. 12J: Plane of nucleus mass and phaco tip should be usually at one level.

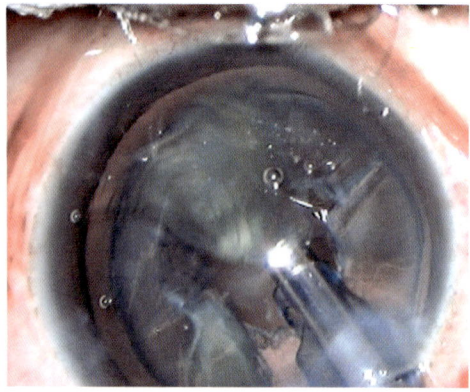

Fig. 12K: Only phaco tip without chopper in the eye for better followability of the tissue which hastens the nucleus emulsification.

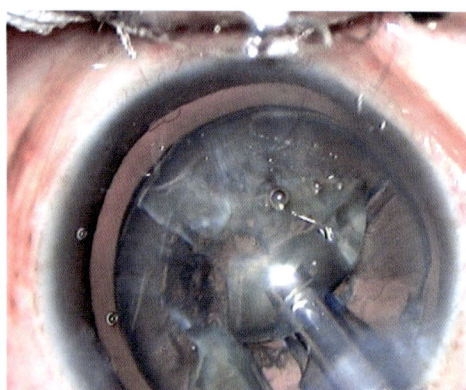

Fig. 12L: Direction of phaco tip toward nucleus mass; bevel-up position of phaco tip for emulsification of nucleus mass is having advantage of better visualization and better fluidics.

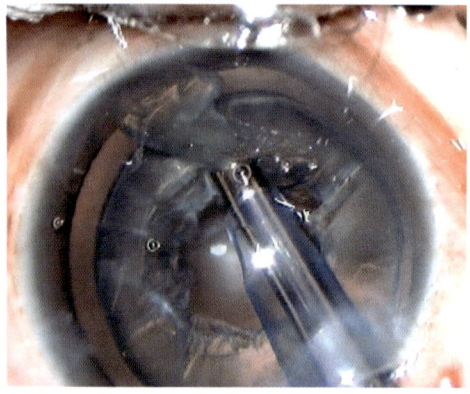

Fig. 12M: The peripheral piece brought at the central safe zone before emulsification.

Removal of Small Pieces of Nucleus

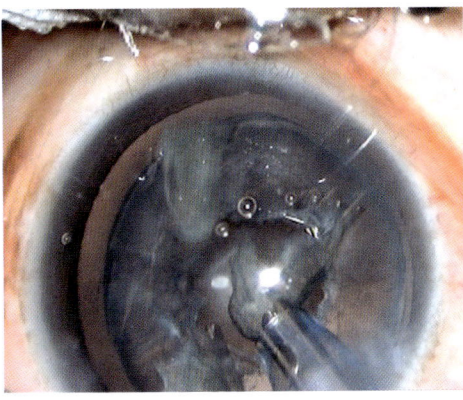

Fig. 12N: For peripheral nucleus piece, do not emulsify the complete nucleus mass at periphery. Only engage the nucleus with minimum energy and bring it to the center and emulsify.

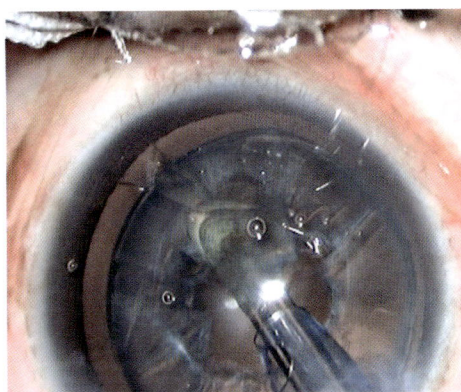

Fig. 12O: Phaco tip usually should not cross 180°.

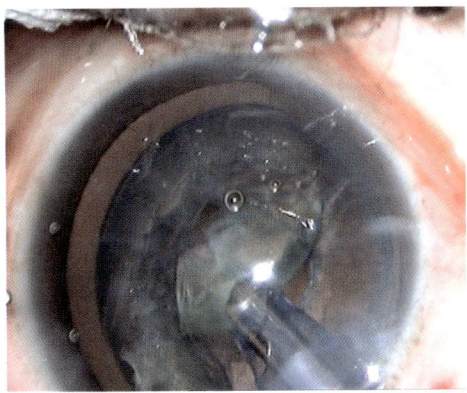

Fig. 12P: Nuclear mass should be horizontal or oriented horizontally before emulsification to avoid mechanical injury to cornea.

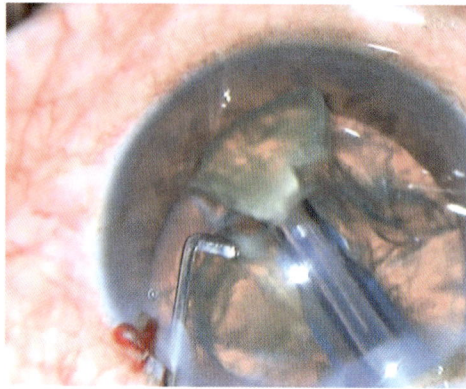

Fig. 12Q: Phaco tip at the apex of nucleus mass will speed up the procedure of removal.

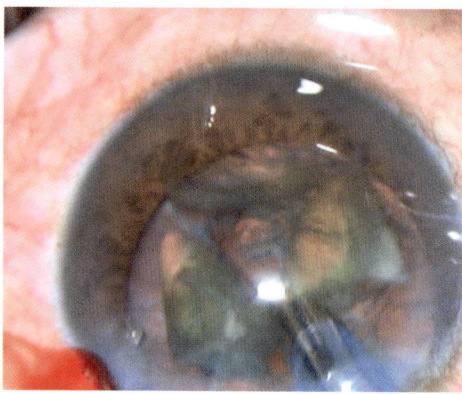

Fig. 12R: During removal of one piece, the other pieces lying in the same plane are easy to remove.

Removal of Small Pieces of Nucleus

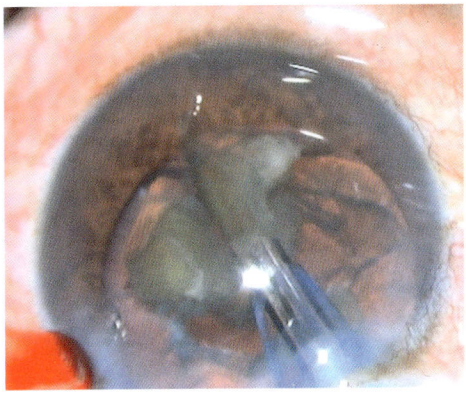

Fig. 12S: Phaco tip directed toward the long axis of the nucleus mass.

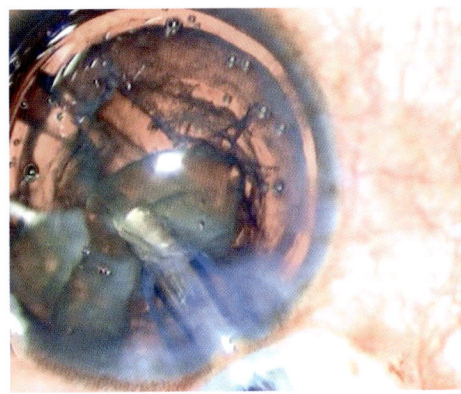

Fig. 12T: Orientation of the phaco tip in such a way that one piece is engaged and at the same time apex of another piece is adjacent to the tip for easy removal.

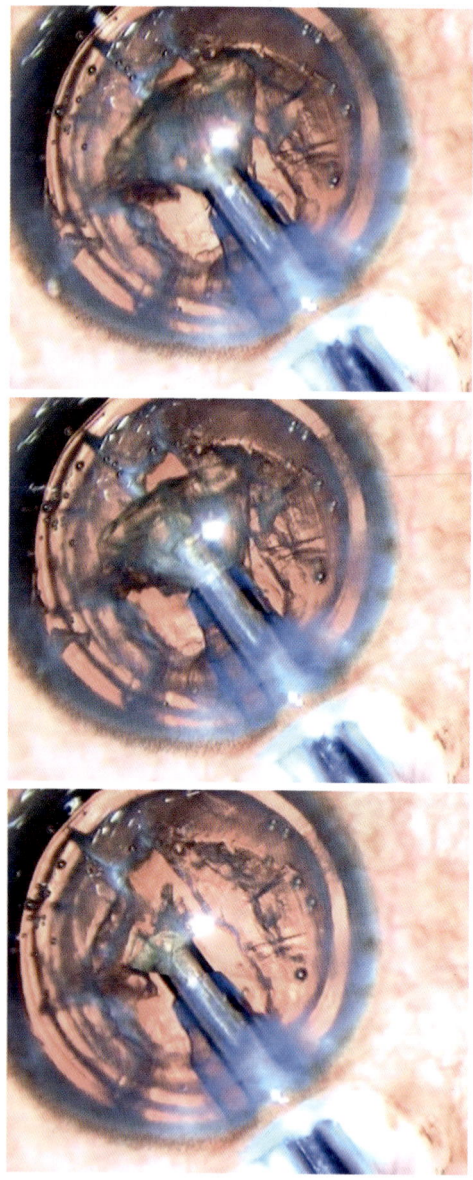

Fig. 12U: During removal of last and small piece, cut down all the parameters.

CHAPTER 13

Irrigation and Aspiration

■ INTRODUCTION

Irrigation and aspiration (I/A) is one of the most important steps in phaco surgery. Posterior capsule rupture (PCR) and zonular dialysis are common during this step.

■ TYPES

- *Manual:* Simcoe cannula
- *Automated:*
  - Coaxial I/A
  - Bimanual I/A

■ COAXIAL IRRIGATION–ASPIRATION

Irrigation and aspiration by one tip is called coaxial I/A. Types of tips are **(Fig. 1)**:
- Straight tip
- 45° tip
- 90° tip

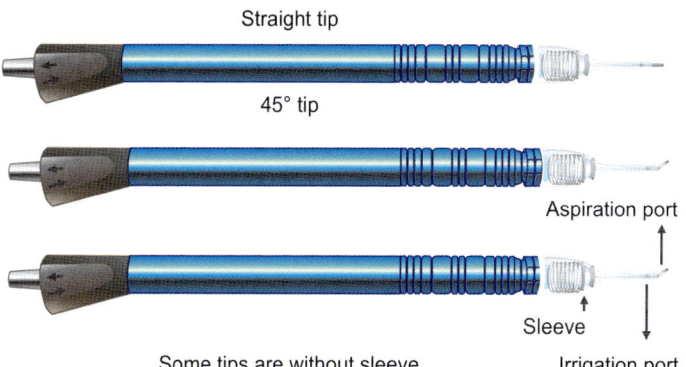

Fig. 1: Coaxial irrigation–aspiration (types of tips).

Irrigation and Aspiration

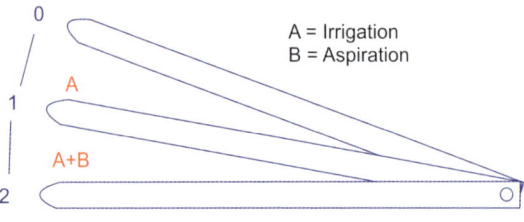

Fig. 2: Foot pedal position.

Design

Coaxial I/A is an automated system. Irrigation is from two sides of the tip 180° apart. Aspiration port is a single aspiration port situated just away from the tip (concave side of the curved tip). The lumen is from 0.2 to 0.7 mm and commonly used is 0.3 mm.

This I/A tip can be with or without sleeve.

Foot Pedal Position (Fig. 2)

This step is used for removal of cortex, epinucleus, and very soft nucleus. Irrigation is continuous and aspiration is under the surgeon's control. It means that foot pedal position 1 is irrigation and foot pedal position 2 is I/A. Soft tissue is the same in all quadrants. Irrigating fluid is helpful to loosen the cortex.

Significance is that PCR and zonular dialysis are common in this step, so to deal with this issue and learning the methodology is very important.

Parameters

Vacuum: 200–350 mm Hg

Aspiration flow rate: 10–20%

Linear mode and gradual rise as per the requirement.

Principles and Some Facts Related to Irrigation–Aspiration (Fig. 3)

- *Aspirate first where there is:*
  - Bulk of the tissue
  - Apex of the tissue
- Always try to go under the hood

Irrigation and Aspiration

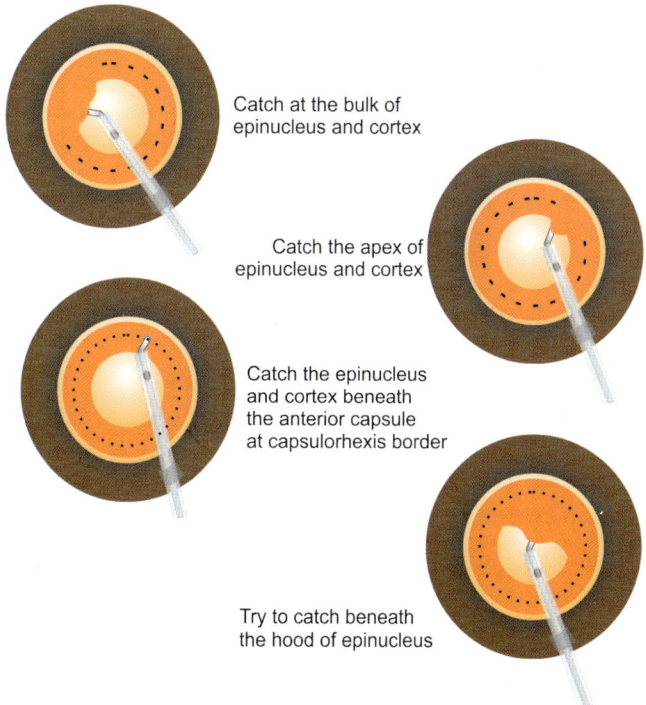

Fig. 3: Principles of irrigation–aspiration.

- Horizontal position of the eye and a good red glow
- Removal of soft tissue should be parallel to structures.
- Try to remove tissue in layers, i.e., epinucleus first followed by cortex.
- Aspiration is done in three zones. To understand aspiration, we will divide the field into three zones.
- Usually, first remove the soft tissue of zone I, then go to zone II, and finally to zone III.

Technique

Check the flow of irrigation and press the foot pedal to position 2; vacuum will not rise. See flow of irrigating fluid and efficacy of aspiration port and setting of machine. Pass the I/A cannula horizontally and place it in the center of the eye and then get the horizontal position. Aspiration port should be always beneath the anterior capsule as soft tissue follows the contour of the capsule.

Irrigation and Aspiration

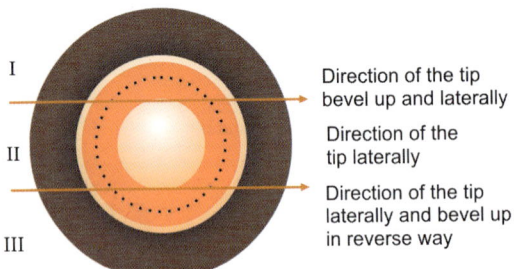

Fig. 4: Direction of irrigation–aspiration tip in different zones.

Aspiration port should always be under visualization. Aspiration should always be directed toward the tissue to be removed.

Direction of Irrigation–Aspiration Tip in Different Zones (Fig. 4)

Direction of I/A port is different in different zones which is a very crucial factor to hasten procedure of I/A and to make this procedure simple and safe.

Procedure of Irrigation–Aspiration (Fig. 5)

Procedure of I/A—removal of soft tissue in I/A usually starts from zone I, zone II, and then zone III. Application of principle and direction of I/A tip is important throughout the procedure.

Significant Points Related to three Zones for Irrigation–Aspiration (Fig. 6)

Aspiration of Soft Tissue in Zone I

Significance: Bevel-up or oblique position of tip is at 6 o'clock and then move the aspiration port of tip in horizontal position toward the bulk laterally.

Advantages:
- Easily accessible
- Better visualization
- Chamber is well formed
- All the structures are apart
- Dilatation of the pupils is maximum
- Phaco fluidics is working better

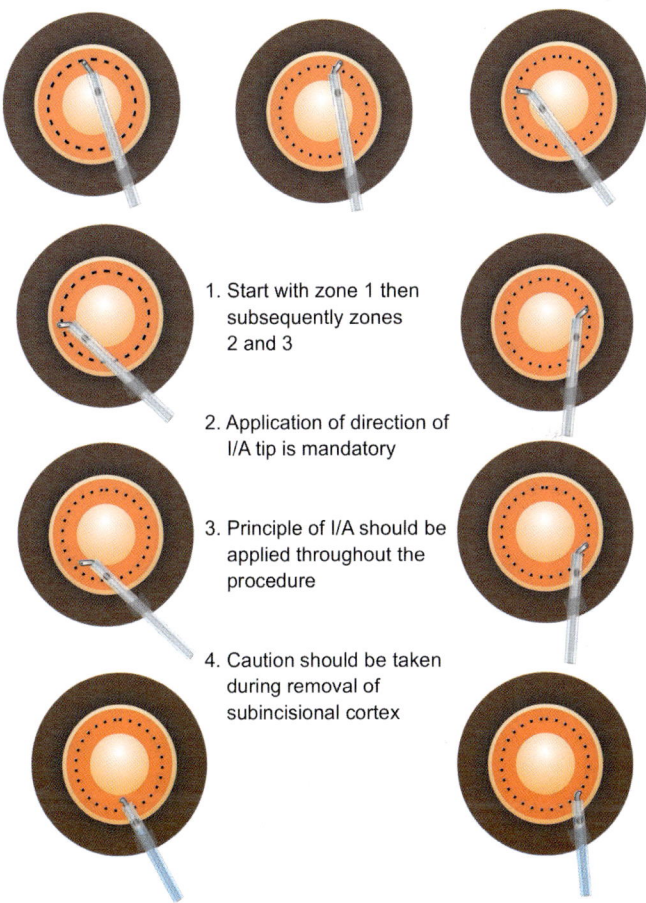

Fig. 5: Procedure of irrigation–aspiration (I/A).

1. Start with zone 1 then subsequently zones 2 and 3
2. Application of direction of I/A tip is mandatory
3. Principle of I/A should be applied throughout the procedure
4. Caution should be taken during removal of subincisional cortex

Aspiration in Zone II

Position of tip is bevel sideways. Most of the cortex in zone II is aspirated in continuity with zone I.

Aspiration in Zone III

It is the most difficult zone as:
- Less visualization
- Poor fluidics as fluid comes out of chamber in this position
- Chamber is not well formed and unstable.
- Putting the instrument is awkward.

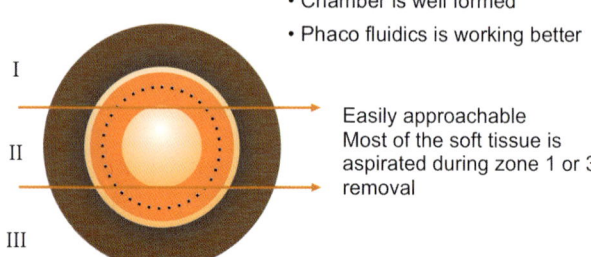

Fig. 6: Significant points related to different zones during I/A zones. (I/A: irrigation and aspiration; PCR: posterior capsule rupture)

- Depending on size of capsulorhexis
- All structures are near to the port.
- More chances of PCR
- The movement of tip during aspiration of tissue should be fast and should bring it toward the center of the eye.

Sometimes, remove the tissue quadrant-wise and preferably keep removing adjacent cortex as there is already a tangential pull to the tissue.

Sometimes, the soft tissue may be sticky, and chopper may be required to touch the aspiration port of I/A tip for easy removal of cortex and epinucleus.

Points to be Avoided During Procedure of Irrigation and Aspiration (Fig. 7)

- Aspiration port should not be directed toward cornea and posterior capsule.
- When I/A tip moves from one point to another side, foot pedal position should be 1 or there should be continuous irrigation only and no aspiration.
- I/A should not be over the hood of soft tissue.

Irrigation and Aspiration   173

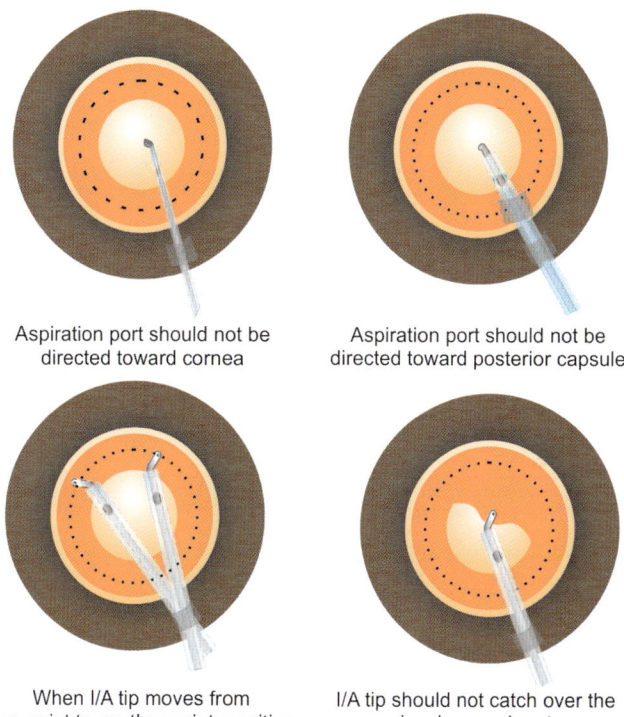

Fig. 7: Point to be avoided during procedure of irrigation–aspiration (I/A).

■ CAP-VAC MODE

- Removing the cells and material from anterior and posterior capsule is called polishing of anterior and posterior capsule.
- *Vacuum:* 5–10 mm Hg
- *Aspiration:* 5–10%

■ COMPLICATIONS

- PCR
- Iris prolapse
- Descemet's membrane detachment
- Avulsion of the bag
- Zonular dialysis
- Iridodialysis

Viscoexpression of Epinucleus and Cortex

Epinucleus and cortex can be easily removed by viscoelastics. Put the visco at 7 o'clock position beneath anterior capsule in the bag to lift epinucleus and cortex from that area. Once this soft tissue comes out, put visco cannula on 4 o'clock to lift that mass. Throughout the procedure, visco cannula is behind the soft tissue, put visco continuously and at the same time press posterior lip of incision to remove soft tissue. This procedure is called viscoexpression of soft tissue. This step will definitely assist further procedure of I/A.

■ BIMANUAL IRRIGATION–ASPIRATION

Definition

- Two different instruments needed—so-called bimanual I/A
- One instrument is needed for irrigation.
- Other instrument is needed for aspiration.

Design (Figs. 8A and B)

- Irrigation handle has two holes sideways, 180° apart for irrigation.
- Aspiration handle has one hole at distal end in bevel-up position for aspiration.

Procedure

Irrigation from one side port and aspiration from other side port with same principles of removal of cortex which has been mentioned already **(Figs. 9 and 10)**.

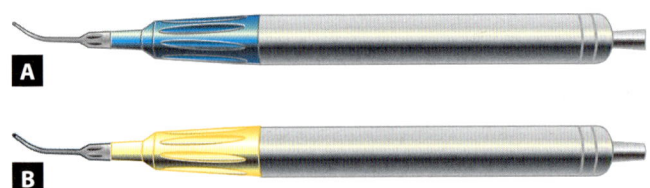

Figs. 8A and B: Bimanual irrigation–aspiration (design): (A) Irrigation cannula and (B) Aspiration cannula.

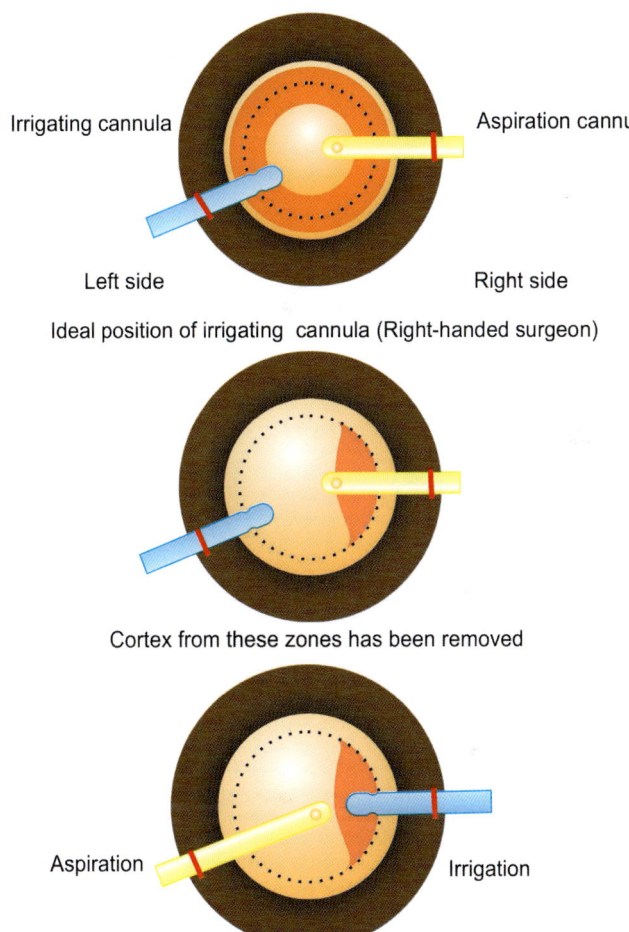

Fig. 9: Position of irrigation-aspiration cannula.

Advantages

- Control on eyeball is better.
- Horizontal position can be maintained during I/A.
- Complete removal of soft tissue 360° is easily possible as I/A cannula can be interchanged through side port.
- 12 o'clock cortex removal is easy.

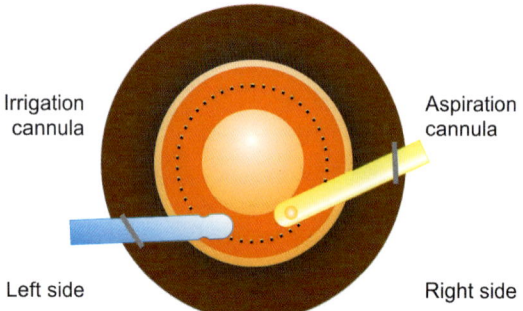
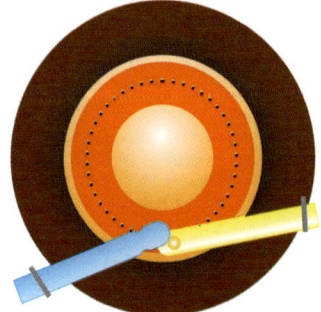

Fig. 10: Advantage of bimanual irrigation-aspiration procedure.

- Sometimes, removal of soft tissue is easy by tucking two instruments to each other when cortex blocks the aspiration port.

Disadvantages
- Two hands are engaged, so there is diversion of mind.
- Sometimes, abnormal pressure occurs on eyeball.
- I/A cannulas are without sleeve, so after procedure, many times there is leakage from side port as incision gets distorted.

MANUAL IRRIGATION AND ASPIRATION
Simcoe Cannula
It is the real form of manual I/A system.

Principle

Irrigation means deepening and creating space and aspiration means removal of soft tissue such as epinucleus–cortex manually.

Technique

Cannula should be passed parallel to posterior capsule via main port or side port. Soft material, which is in vicinity or propped out of the bag, should be removed first and then remove the tissue in the periphery of the bag.

Precaution

Check the flow of irrigation cannula before inserting it inside the eye.

■ INDICATIONS IN PHACO

- Learning stage of automated I/A
- Continuous iris prolapse during coaxial I/A
- Runaway of capsulorhexis
- During leaky wound in I/A
- Improper wound construction
- Floppy iris syndrome
- Small pupil
- Removal of subincisional cortex in small continuous curvilinear capsulorhexis through side port incision.

■ COMPLICATIONS

- Injury to corneal endothelium
- Iris prolapses
- Iridodialysis with subsequent hyphema
- Zonular dialysis
- PCR
- PCR with zonular dialysis with vitreous loss

■ KEY POINTS

- This is one of the most important steps to be learned gradually as PCR and zonular dialysis are very common during this step.

- Start with manual Simcoe cannula and then shift to automated I/A system.
- Direction of aspiration port toward mass is the most important factor.
- One should know about reflux before the start of automated I/A system.

■ LIVE SURGERY PHOTOGRAPHS (FIGS. 11A TO R)

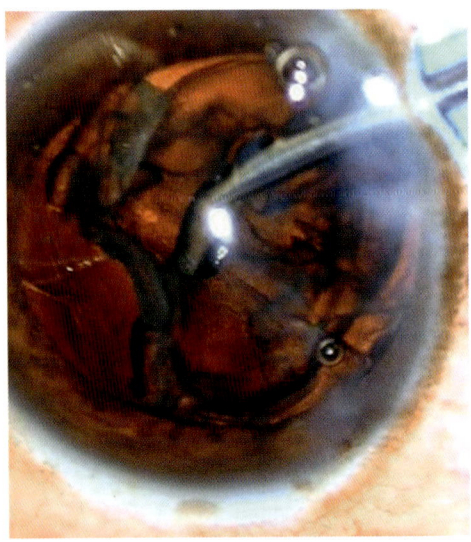

Fig. 11A: Placement of irrigation–aspiration canula is horizontal. Catching the apex of soft tissue.

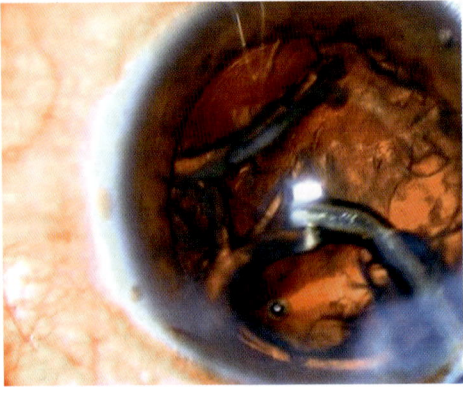

Fig. 11B: Removal of epinucleus under visualization.

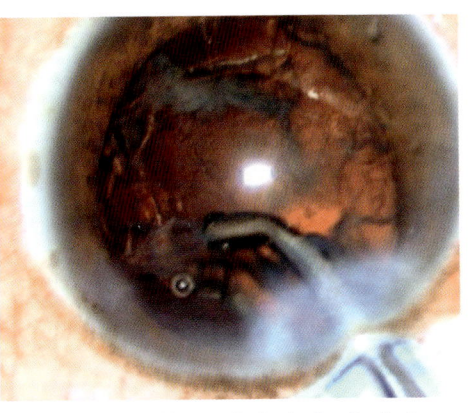

Fig. 11C: Preferably, catch the bulk of soft tissue.

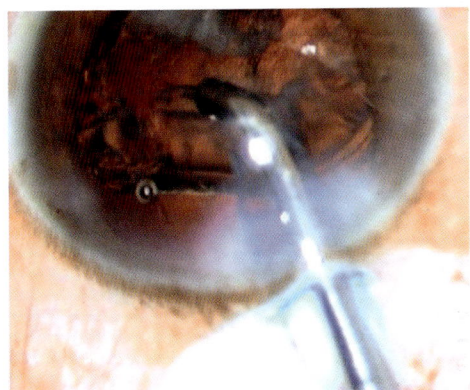

Fig. 11D: Lifting of subincisional cortex, by keeping the irrigation–aspiration tip vertically down under observation.

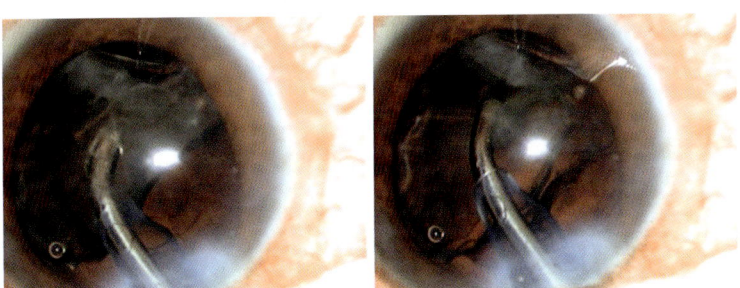

Fig. 11E: Removal of tissue by catching the epinucleus sheet under the hood.

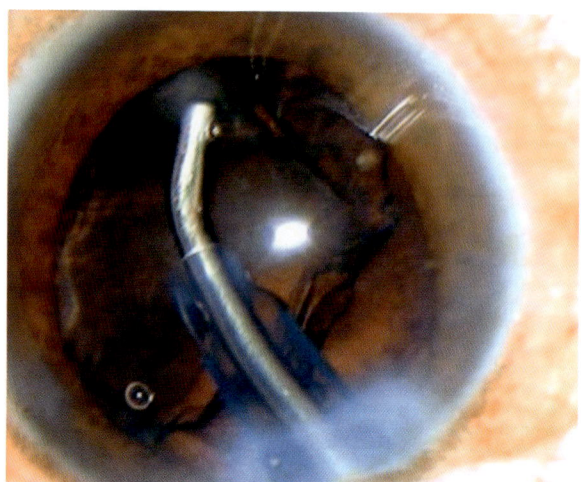

Fig. 11F: At 6 o'clock position, soft tissue catchment with tilted bevel-up position.

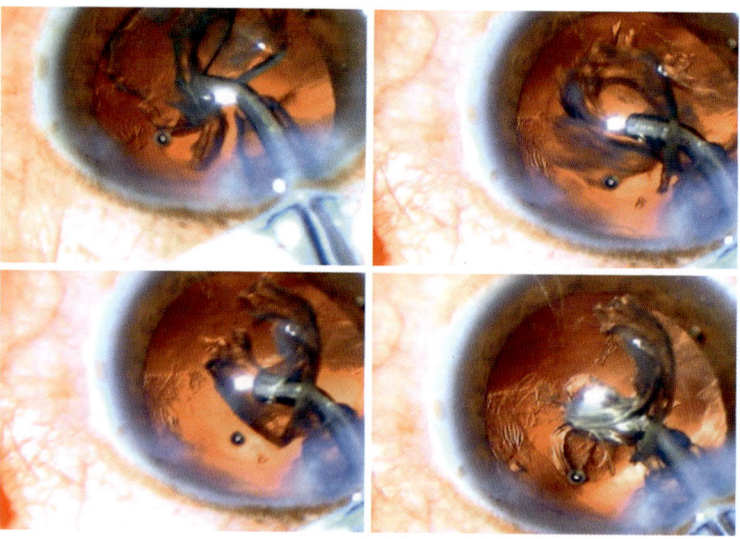

Fig. 11G: Once the edge of epinucleus is caught, aspiration is very fast.

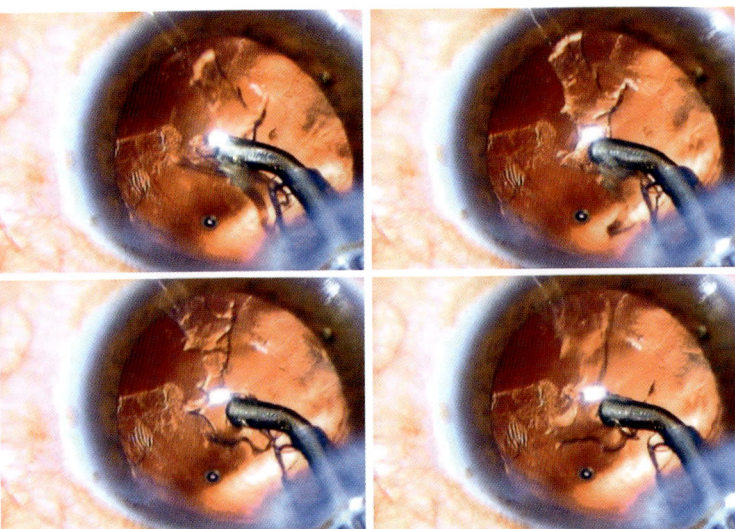

Fig. 11H: Epinucleus sheet removed with horizontal placement of irrigation–aspiration tip in the center.

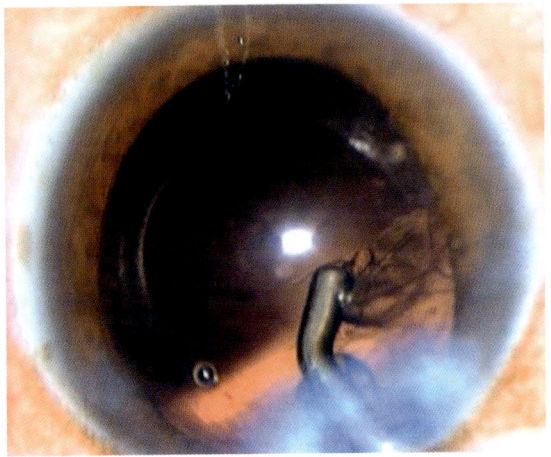

Fig. 11I: 9 o'clock position soft tissue caught by placing irrigation–aspiration cannula in bevel sideway position.

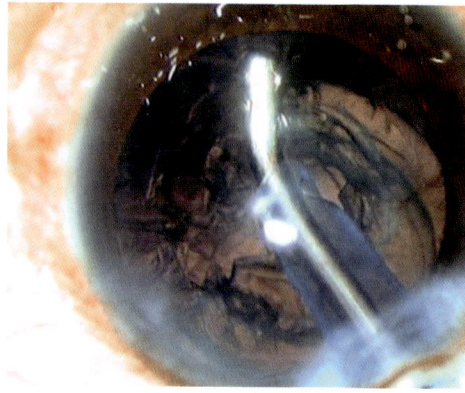

Fig. 11J: Start the irrigation–aspiration at 6 o'clock position, which assists dislodgment of the soft tissue from other clock hours easily.

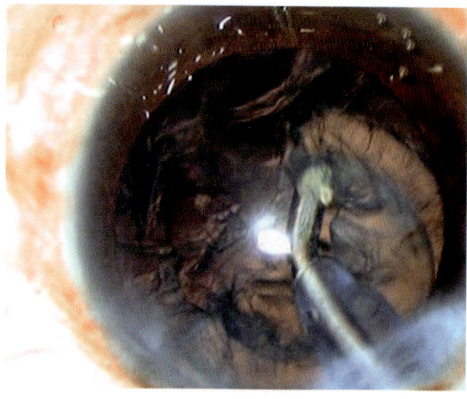

Fig. 11K: Other preferable sites of aspiration are bulk of soft tissue from the edge.

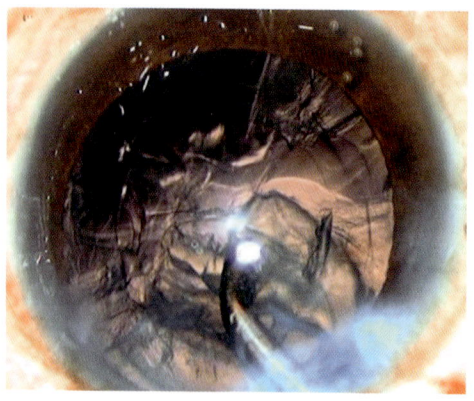

Fig. 11L: Usually, remove the epinucleus before cortex. Here, by placing the irrigation–aspiration cannula under the hood.

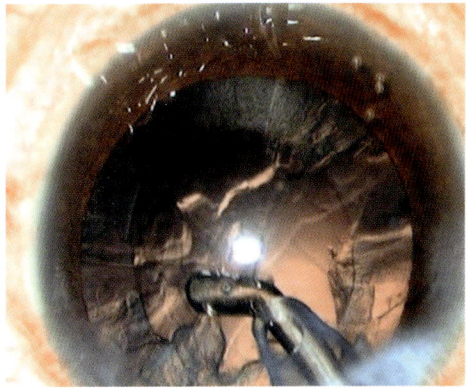

Fig. 11M: Remaining epinucleus sheet removed by catching the apex.

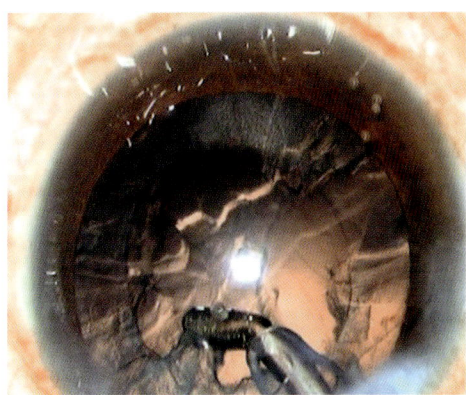

Fig. 11N: Apex and bulk from 1 o'clock position aspirated.

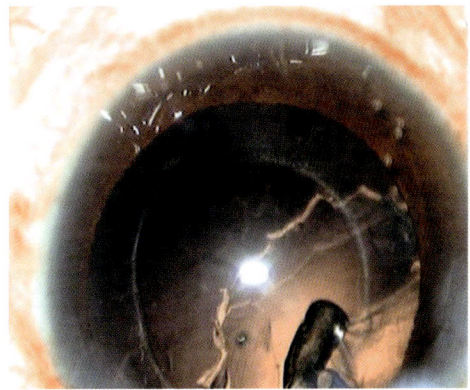

Fig. 11O: Finally, thin sheet of cortex is aspirated.

Figures 11P1 to P5—Clockwise Removal of Soft Tissue

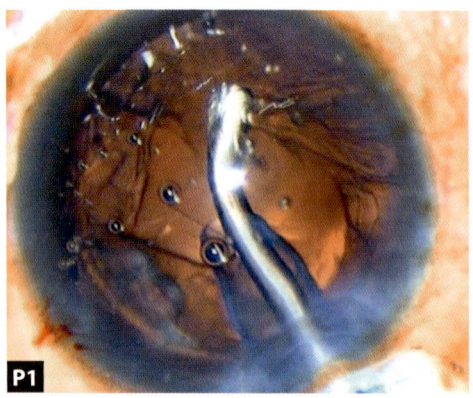

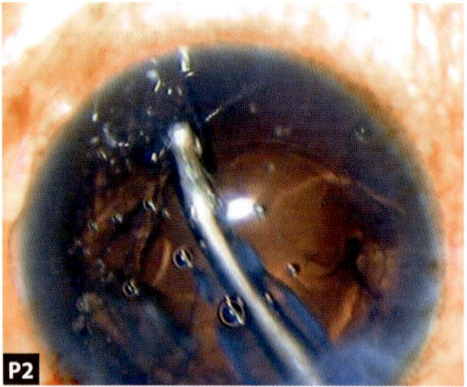

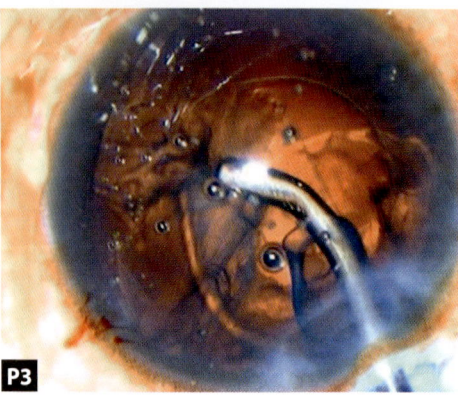

Figs. 11P1 to P3: (P1) 9 o'clock position of soft tissue: Catching by bevel sideways position of irrigation–aspiration cannula and catching the apex; (P2) 6 o'clock position of soft tissue: Catching by bevel-up or bevel oblique position; (P3) 3 o'clock position by keeping direction of aspiration port toward the mass. Bulk of the tissue should aspirate preferably.

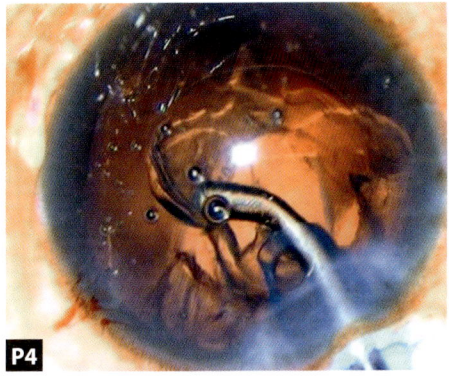

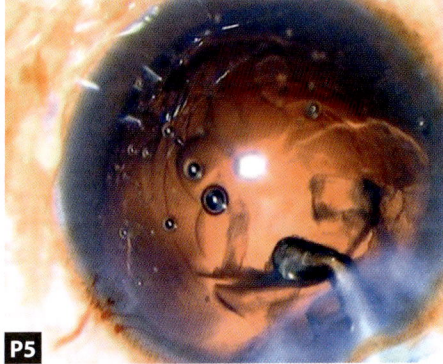

Figs. 11P4 and P5: (P4) 1 o'clock position by keeping the probe horizontally, remove the epinucleus first and then cortex; (P5) At 12 o'clock position sub-incisional cortex can be removed under visualization, maintaining anterior chamber, catching of tissue with bevel down position and aspiration with bevel sideway position towards center.

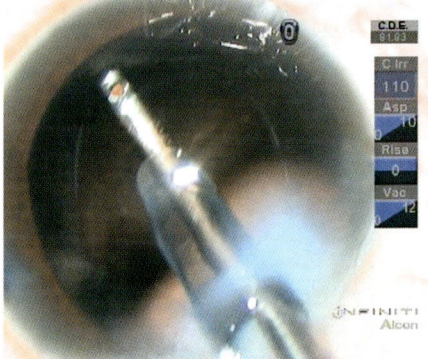

Fig. 11Q: Anterior subcapsular polish with irrigation–aspiration cannula by minimum vacuum and flow rate.

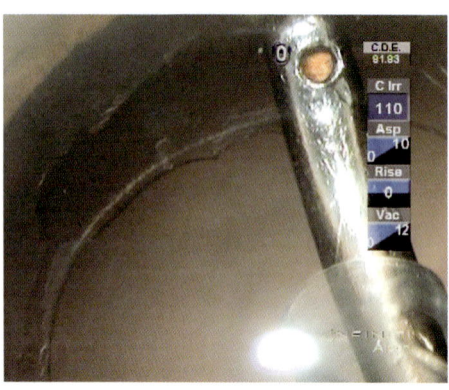

Fig. 11R: Polishing and removal of cells seen under higher magnification.

Intraocular Lens: Basic and Technical Aspects

CHAPTER 14

INTRODUCTION
- An opacity in the lens or in capsule is called cataract.
- Surgical procedure is needed to remove cataract.
- There are various methods of cataract extraction such as phacoemulsification, small-incision cataract surgery (SICS), and extracapsular cataract extraction (ECCE). The removal of cloudy natural lens should be replaced by an artificial lens inside the eye which is called intraocular lens (IOL) implant.

MATERIALS USED
- *Polymethyl methacrylate (PMMA):* It is a plastic material.
- *Silicone lenses:* This lens is made of silicone material.
- *Hydrophilic acrylic:* Water content of this lens is more; this is soft material.
- *Hydrophobic acrylic:* There is no water content in this lens; this material is hard and tough.
- *Heparin surface-modified lens:* Any lens which is coated with heparin is called heparin surface-modified lens.

TYPES OF IOLs
- *Foldable:*
    - Silicone
    - Hydrophilic acrylic
    - Hydrophobic acrylic
- *Nonfoldable:*
    - PMMA

Design of IOLs—Related to Structure
- *Three-piece lenses:*
    - Optic and haptic are of different material; color is also different.

- Optic may be PMMA or hydrophobic acrylic
- Haptic is polypropylene.
- *Single-piece lens:* Optic and haptic are of same material.

Shape of IOLs

- Optic with two haptic
- Optic with three haptic
- Optic with four haptic
- Plate haptic IOL.

Size of IOLs

- Optic size varies from 5.00 to 6.50 mm and overall length varies from 12.00 to 13.50 mm in length.
- Four-petal design lens size is around 10.00 mm.

DIFFERENT CLASSIFICATION

- *Monofocal:* Single focal point
- *Multifocal:* Multiple focal points. Multiple segments are there to see at various distances from near to far objects.
- *Toric lens:* To correct corneal astigmatism
- *Accommodative lens* can give accommodative effect inside the eye.
- *Heparin surface-modified lens:* Used in diabetic patients and uveitic patients (postinflammatory cataract).
- *Advance monofocal lens:* Distant and intermediate vision.
- *Extended depth of focus (EDOF):* Focal segment to give distance and intermediate depth of vision.

OTHER CLASSIFICATION

Primary IOL: IOL put at the same time after cataract extraction procedure.

Secondary IOL: IOL put at later stage after cataract extraction that is in aphakic eyes.

FOLDABLE IOLs

This IOL can be folded while putting inside, then it opens to resume its original shape.

Advantages
- Can go through small incision
- Early rehabilitation of patients
- Posterior capsule opacification (PCO) chances are less.

Technique to put Foldable Intraocular Lens
There are two methods to put foldable IOL:
1. Holder and Folder method
2. Injector system

Principles
- Placement of lens should be parallel to iris and anterior and posterior capsule.
- Putting of IOL should be very slow as each lens, cartridge, and lens with cartridge behaves differently.

Holder and Folder method
- Simple method to put IOL
- Need of special forceps for this method
- Extension of size of incision is needed to put the IOL by this technique.
- This was popular technique or only technique before injectors were introduced in the market.
- Nowadays, rarely, this technique is applied in practice or advised.

Injector system
Every foldable lens has its own cartridge for loading of lens. It should be practiced and mastered by taking help of technical people. After successful loading of lens, placement of foldable IOL with cartridge is real surgeon's work.

Cartridge: Check the cartridge first to check for any manufacturing defect. See for distal end of cartridge related to design, size, and shape for its correlation with incision.

Injector: Nondisposable injector should be checked before use. Disposable injectors should be checked for its movement and spring action. Also, check if there is any match or mismatch between injector and cartridge.

Loading of lens: Different lenses have different techniques to load the lens. Perfect loading of lens should be learned by technicians.

Procedure: After checking everything, lens is loaded along with cartridge and injector is ready to put. Incision should always be adequate sized. Eyeball should be in primary position. Once cartridge is in the center, start pushing injector. Lens will come out of injector slowly. At this point, place the injector little back and leading haptic should be in the bag, then part of optic also should go in the bag; procedure should be slow and completely under our own visualization. Once optic is in the bag, slowly pass trailing haptic in the bag. Always confirm that IOL is in the bag or not.

Thing that can Happen During Foldable Intraocular Lens Implantation

- Injury to corneal epithelium
- Descemet's membrane detachment
- Difficulty to put IOL through incision so that IOL can fall out of eye
- Sometimes, optic or haptic part of IOL trapped in incision
- Optic or haptic part of IOL can be broken mainly at the junction of optic and haptic or distal end of haptic.
- Injury to corneal endothelium, iris, or capsule can occur.
- Placement of IOL is not in bag or partially in bag and partially in sulcus.
- Crack in optics or haptic
- Zonular dialysis
- Posterior capsule rupture (PCR)
- Sometimes, placement of IOL can be in reverse fashion.
  Procedure of putting foldable IOL should be very slow to avoid all these happenings and complications associated with it.

Difficulties or Relative Contraindications for Foldable Intraocular Lens

- If intraoperative complication such as PCR occurs
- If AC or bag is shallow which is noticed during surgery
- If there is positive pressure intraoperatively.

■ POLYMETHYL METHACRYLATE LENS

Advantages
- Can be put after SICS or ECCE
- Cost is less
- This lens can be considered after PCR
- Sometimes in shallow AC, shallow bag, or in intraoperative positive pressure cases.

Technique to put Polymethyl Methacrylate Lens
- AC is to be filled with viscoelastic solution.
- First, check the IOL under microscope related to manufacturing defects.
- Wash the lens anteriorly and posteriorly by balanced salt solution (BSS)
- Hold the lens on the superior aspect of optic by McPherson forcep.
- Placement of the lens inside AC should be parallel to iris.
- First, leading haptic should be in the bag, then optic, then catch trailing haptic and rotate clockwise and at the same time haptic directed posteriorly behind iris and then perfect placement of trailing haptic and optic in the bag
- Most important thing is that placement of IOL should be parallel to iris and posterior capsule throughout the procedure.
- Sometimes, dialer can be used to rotate the lens to put in proper position.

Difficult Situation to put Polymethyl Methacrylate Intraocular Lens
- Deep socket
- Iris prolapsed during procedure.

■ FINISHING STEPS OF PHACO SURGERY AFTER PUTTING INTRAOCULAR LENS

Removal of viscoelastics from AC, bag and behind IOL to be done by irrigation-aspiration cannula.

By irrigating cannula, important things to be noticed are to:
- Check remaining cortex.
- Check for hyphema and iris pigment dispersal.
- Check for placement of IOL.
- Check for wound leak through incision ports.
- Check for stability and pressure of AC.
- See for foreign bodies such as cotton particle, conjunctival tags, and green thread.
- At the end, remove the speculum carefully.

■ KEY POINTS
- Putting foldable IOL should be very slow.
- Practice of loading of lens is very important which varies with different IOL.

CHAPTER 15

No Hydro in Phaco

■ INTRODUCTION

- The author has started phaco surgery in 1997. During initial cases of phaco surgery also, there was not much significance of rotation of nucleus before trench in stop and chop technique of phaco. Theory behind this was that any round or oval mass (nucleus) in a round or oval space will rotate (bag), and so there is no need to check this rotation. As hydro procedures promoted for this rotation, the author did minimum hydroprocedures.
- Secondly, concepts of no or minimum hydro with no rotation were getting confirmed when the author had started phaco training program in 2002. Doctors who were coming for training in phaco, one of the most difficult steps which the author found was hydroprocedures and rotation of the nucleus before trench in their surgical hand.
- Training program at Navneet Hospital, Solapur mainly concentrates on nucleus management steps which include:
  - Trench
  - Division of nucleus
  - Hold and chop in one hemisphere
  - Emulsification of small pieces
  - Repeat procedure for the other hemisphere

    The author feels that the most important step among all is "trench and division of nucleus." Most important prerequisite for trench is immobile nucleus and on the contrary by doing hydro and rotation, we make nucleus mobile. So, this was the third point when author felt that hydroprocedures should be reduced or avoided.
- Training is the best learning process for the author also and now he feels that hydro and rotation of nucleus may give undue stress and force on zonules and weaken the bag, so it is better to avoid

such procedures and further complications—this was the fourth point of thinking.
- Today is the era of premium lenses such as multifocal, toric, multifocal with toric advance monofocal and EDOF lenses which needs a more stable bag and zonules for better performance of lenses and visual outcome, thus thinking of no hydro is becoming more prominent in the author's mind.

■ DEFINITION

Hydroprocedures (Fig. 1)

Hydroprocedures are used for separation of layers of the lens by fluid. Different hydroprocedures are as follows:
- *Hydrodelineation*: Separation between inner hard core of nucleus and adjacent epinucleus
- *Hydrodelamination*: Separation of lens at different zones of epinucleus
- *Hydrodissection*: Separation of cortex and capsule

Advantages of Hydroprocedures
- Rotation of nucleus is easy.
- Less stress on zonules during lens management and easy irrigation aspiration of epinucleus and cortex (conventional approach)

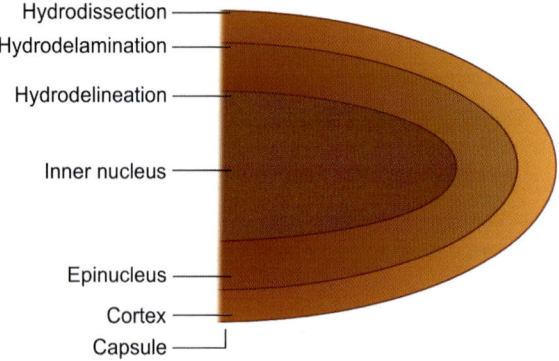

Fig. 1: Exact location of different hydroprocedure.

EVOLUTION OF PHACO SURGERY IN AUTHOR'S PRACTICE RELATED TO HYDROPROCEDURES

Stop and Chop Technique

- *Initial days (1997-2002):* After capsulorhexis, hydrodelineation and hydrodissection were done in all the cases, but no rotation of nucleus before trench.
- *After some days (2003-2007):* Hydrodelineation only in indicated cases and no hydrodissection
- *Today (2008 onward):* No hydroprocedures except for very soft cataract (Grade I)

Surgical Techniques

- Incision
- Capsulorhexis
- No hydrodissection in any case (except very soft cataract and Grade 1 nucleus)
- No rotation before trench, so trench on immobile nucleus
- Division of the nucleus into two pieces
- Hold and chop of one hemisphere and then emulsification of small pieces
- Hold and chop of the other hemisphere and then emulsification of small pieces
- Viscoexpression of epinucleus in indicated cases
- Irrigation and aspiration of epinucleus and cortex
- Foldable intraocular lens (IOL) implantation

While trenching, due to irrigation-effective hydroprocedures are going on, so there is no need for intentional hydroprocedures **(Fig. 2)**.

Overall advantages of no hydro in phaco surgery:
- No unnecessary intrabag manipulation so that no stress on zonules and bag
- Trench on immobile nucleus is easy
- No disturbance of soft tissue; thus, visualization is better
- No increase in intrabag pressure

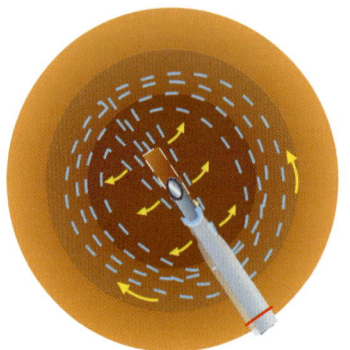

Fig. 2: Hydroprocedure during trench.

While trenching, due to irrigation-effective hydroprocedures are going on, so there is no need of intentional hydroprocedures

- Less chances of capsulolenticular block which is the most dreaded complication

Common indications for no hydro phaco surgery are as follows:
- *Mature cataract:* Since the visualization of different layers of lens is difficult
- *Pseudoexfoliation:* Suspicious zonular weakness
- *Hard cataract*: Space between anterior capsule and nucleus is less.
- *Shallow anterior chamber:* Hydroprocedures can cause anterior chamber to become more shallower.
- *Hazy cornea*: Hydro can further hamper visualization.
- Suspicious zonular weakness like wrinkling on face of patient
- *Posterior polar cataract:* Posterior capsule is weak in center, so chances of PCR during hydro.
- *Subluxated cataract:* Zonular weakness can increase.
- *Small pupil:* With intrabag manipulation, pupillary size can get reduced.

CONCLUSION

By avoiding hydroprocedures, we get the following benefits:
- Surgical steps cut down
- Phaco procedure becomes cleaner and simpler
- Duration of surgery is reduced

- Minimum stress on bag and zonules
- Respect to anatomy is maintained
- Surgical complications are reduced
- Result of premium lenses is better

KEY POINTS
- Intrabag manipulation is reduced due to no hydro technique.
- No hydro phaco surgery has changed the scenario of phaco practice and is a choice of surgery by author.

Finishing Steps in Phacoemulsification Surgery

CHAPTER 16

■ INTRODUCTION

- It is simple but most important step in phaco surgery.
- Removal of viscoelastics thoroughly from anterior segment after implanting intraocular lens (IOL)
- This step is very significant to avoid postoperative complications, such as uveitis and transient rise in IOP, related to the viscoelastics left behind after operation.
- This step is a checkpoint to ensure IOL in situ, central round pupil and IOP of eye.

According to the author, it is an art to do this finishing step of cataract surgery. This step is based on certain principles of physics.

■ PROCEDURE

A: Viscoelastics are removed by irrigation-aspiration (I/A) cannula (bimanual or coaxial).

During removal of viscoelastics from anterior segment, tap IOL with coaxial I/A cannula. Start from center with its full preset value, then move the cannula to periphery up to the edge of iris with decreased parameters. Some surgeons go behind IOL also very gently to remove viscoelastics with minimum parameters.

B: Irrigation with 5cc and 2cc syringe and cannula with BSS
- This is an important step after I/A of viscoelastics.
- With 5cc syringe irrigation is done over the iris in anterior chamber, where direction of cannula is tangential and at the same time posterior lip of incision should be pressed to remove excess BSS.
- This maneuver, helps to remove visco behind the cornea.
- Irrigation is done 360°, all around in the bag to check for remaining cortex. Also it helps in loosening of cortex.

- Finally remove visco from behind the IOL.
- Formation of anterior chamber by putting BSS through side port incision.
- Hydration of incisions may be needed.

COMPLICATIONS
- Iris Prolapse
- Descemet membrane detachment

To avoid iris prolapse
- Tapping of IOL gently during this step.
- Direction of cannula should not be perpendicular to the main incision.
- Adequate pressure on iris is needed many times during this procedure

To avoid Descemet membrane detachment
- Direction of the cannula should not be in the deeper layers of cornea during hydration.

SIGNIFICANCE
- Removal of viscoelastic
- To check whether IOL is in the bag. If IOL rotates freely in bag, it indicates that the IOL is in situ. This checkpoint is important for postoperative results.
- Removal of remaining cortex
- Removal of small, hidden nuclear pieces or cortex which is not easily removed in cases such as hypotony, high myopia, mature cataract, etc.
- Removal of foreign body or debris
- One should check all entries such as main incision and all side port incisions, to look for cortex, nucleus pieces, foreign body, etc.

When to Stop
- Anterior chamber is well formed.
- Anterior chamber should be clear.

- Normotensive eyeball
- Well-centered round pupil

■ KEY POINTS

- This is one of the most important step in phaco surgery.
- Though simple, but this step has a steeper learning curve.
- It is an art to do this step.

CHAPTER 17: Instruments for Phaco Surgery

Instruments needed for phaco surgery are shown in **Figures 1 to 29**.

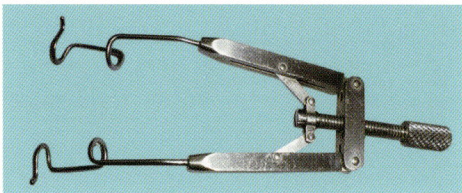

Fig. 1: Speculum.

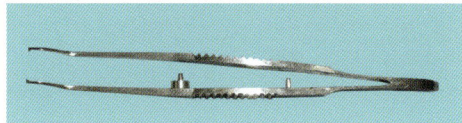

Fig. 2: Superior and inferior rectus forceps.

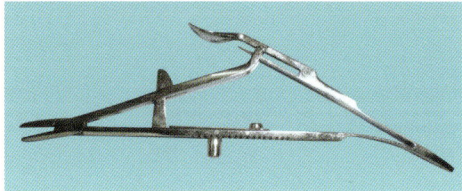

Fig. 3: Silcocks needle holder.

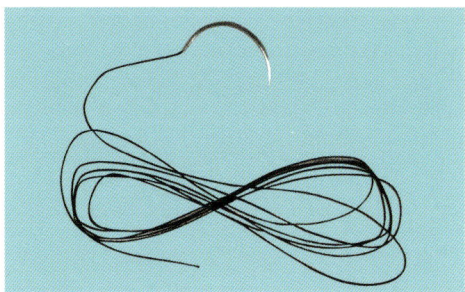

Fig. 4: Needle with white or black thread.

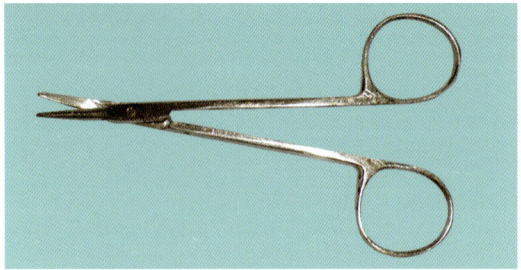

Fig. 5: Curved scissor with blunt edge.

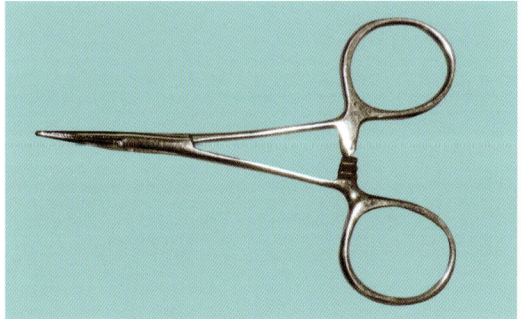

Fig. 6: Artery forcep.

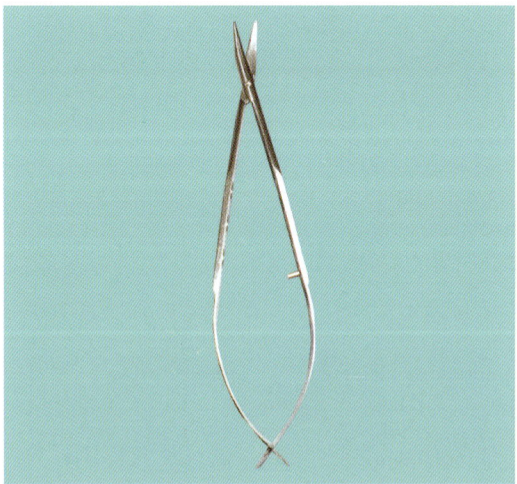

Fig. 7: Conjunctival scissor.

Instruments for Phaco Surgery

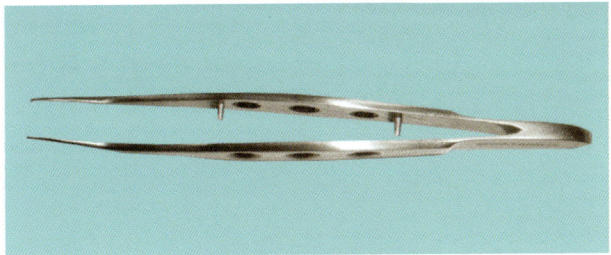

Fig. 8: Tooth forcep.

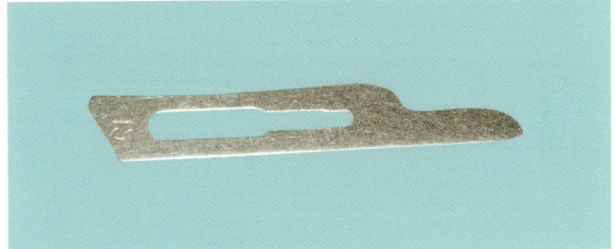

Fig. 9: No. 15 blade.

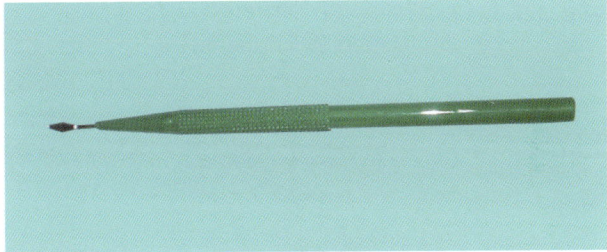

Fig. 10: Crescent.

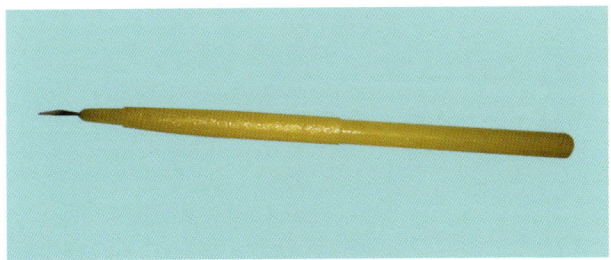

Fig. 11: Side port 15°.

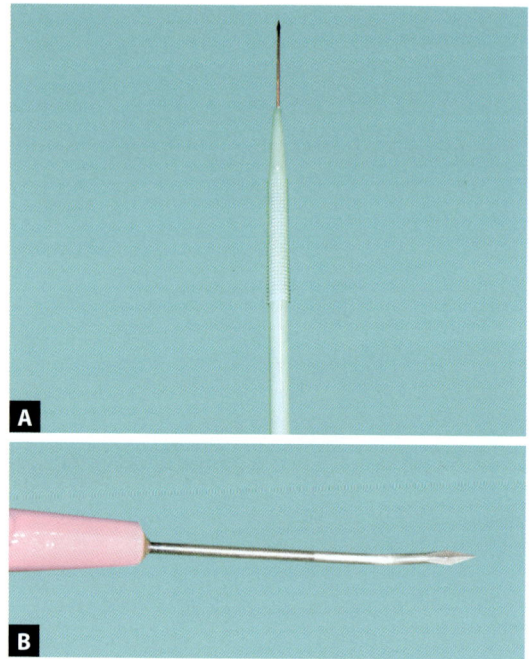

Figs. 12A and B: (A) Side-port microvitreoretinal (MVR) blade; (B) Side-port MVR blade angled.

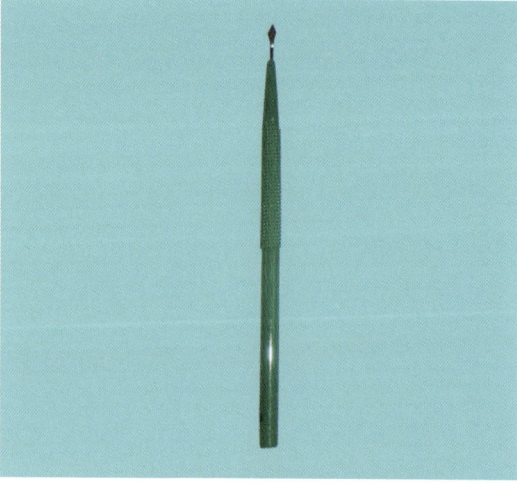

Fig. 13: Keratome (2.00–2.8 mm).

Instruments for Phaco Surgery

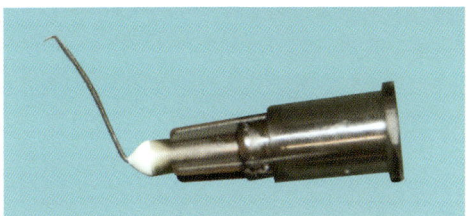

Fig. 14: Cystitome No. 26 needle.

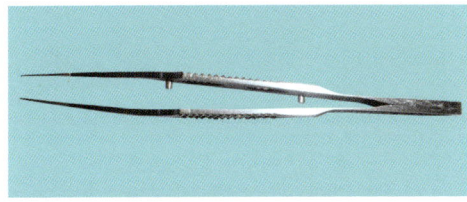

Fig. 15: Capsulorhexis forceps (Utrata).

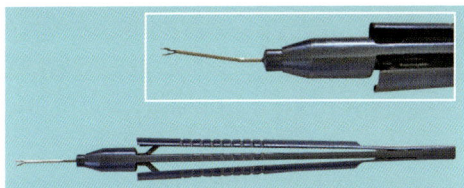

Fig. 16: Toshniwal microcapsulorhexis forcep.

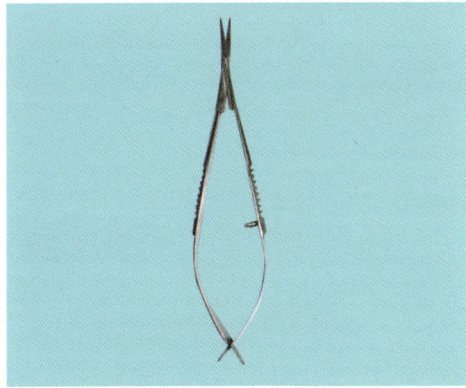

Fig. 17: Vannas scissor.

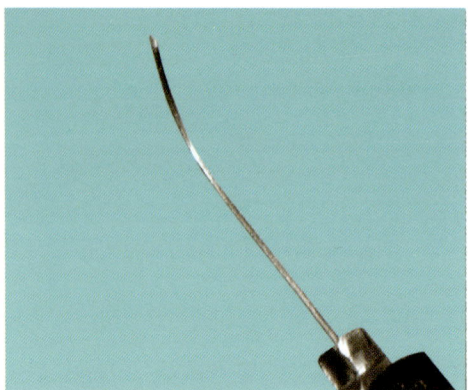

Fig. 18: Hydrodissection cannula.

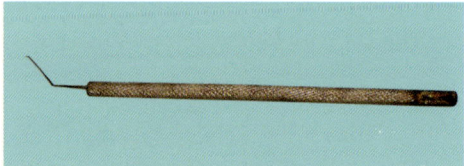

Fig. 19: Dialer.

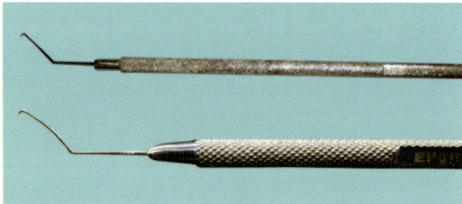

Fig. 20: Chopper.

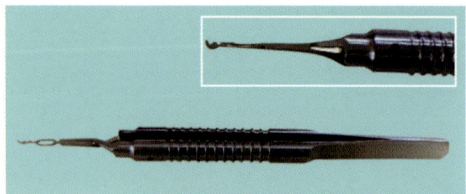

Fig. 21: Toshniwal prechopper.

Instruments for Phaco Surgery

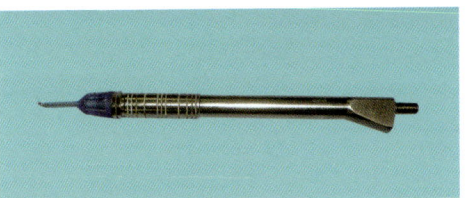

Fig. 22: Coaxial irrigation–aspiration cannula.

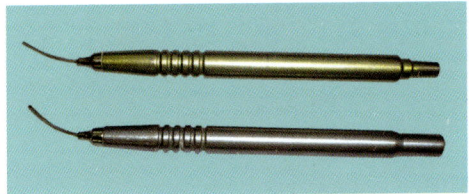

Fig. 23: Bimanual irrigation–aspiration cannula.

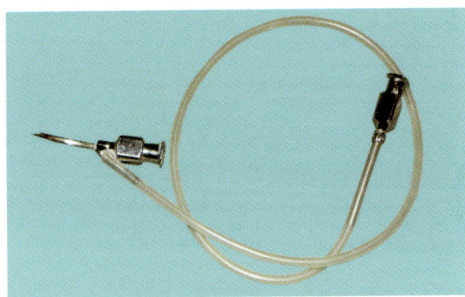

Fig. 24: Simcoe cannula.

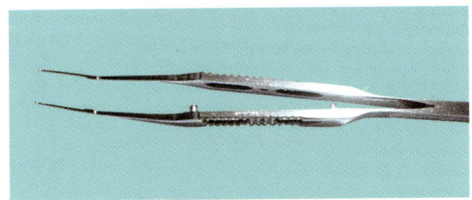

Fig. 25: McPherson forcep.

Instruments for Phaco Surgery

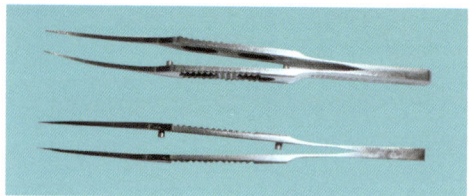

Fig. 26: Suture tying forceps (straight and curved forceps).

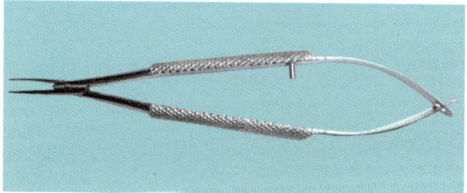

Fig. 27: Spring needle holder.

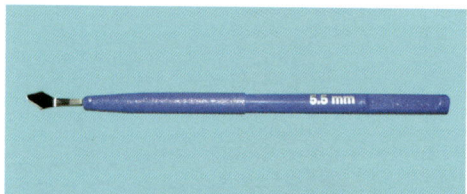

Fig. 28: 5.5 mm keratome.

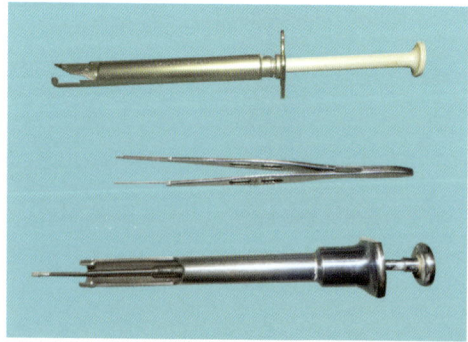

Fig. 29: Injectors for foldable intraocular lens (IOL).

Index

Page numbers followed by *f* refer to figure and *t* refer to table.

A

Adrenaline 34
Air bubble 62
    formation 90
Akahoshi prechopper 103, 103*f*, 107
ALCON legion machine,
        console of 19*f*
Allergy, drugs 8
Alpha-crystallin proteins 3
Anesthesia, types of 34
    general 34, 35, 37
    local 34
    regional 36
    topical 34-36
Angulated blade 48
Anterior capsular 11, 60
    tear 133, 135
Anterior chamber 81, 117*f*, 199
    depth 9
    entry in 45
    maintained 118*f*
    pressure, high 57
    shallow 9, 42, 70, 89, 196
Anterior subcapsular polish 185*f*
Apex and bulk 183*f*
Arcus 46
Artery forcep 202*f*
Aspiration bypass system tip 24
Aspiration cannula 174*f*
Aspiration flow rate 31, 80, 125, 126,
        147, 150
Asthma 6

B

Bag, avulsion of 173
Balanced salt solution 26, 75
Ball and socket 2
Basement membrane, anterior
        capsule with 56*f*
Biconvex crystalline structure 1

Bimanual irrigation aspiration 41, 174
    cannula 207*f*
    procedure, advantage of 176*f*
Blunt edge, curved scissor with 202*f*
Body, texture of 6
Burst mode 30

C

Caliber 46
Capsular
    bag 77
    rent, posterior 135
Capsulolenticular block 77, 78*f*, 79*f*
    chances of 196
Capsulorhexis 10, 39, 41, 56, 58, 61, 65*f*,
        66*f*, 66-68, 71, 79*f*, 89, 93*f*
    choice of solution for 70
    forceps 58, 61, 65*f*, 205*f*
    level of 160*f*
    margin 67
    physics of 57, 58*f*
    practice 71
    prerequisite for 57*f*
    runaway of 71, 72*f*, 177
    speed of 67, 68*f*
    technique of 63, 65*f*
    work of 59
    zones of 66
CAP-VAC mode 173
Cartridge 189
Cataract
    anterior subcapsular 15*f*
    differentiate layers of 18*f*
    for phaco, mature 18*f*
    hard 14*f*, 88, 196
    in vitrectomized eyes 89
    mature 7, 12, 18*f*, 70, 196
    posterior
        polar 12, 196
        subcapsular 7, 16*f*
    pseudoexfoliation 89

soft 7, 88, 112*f*, 134
    division in 111, 112*f*
sticky 7, 134
surgeries 37
variations of trench in different types of 88
very hard 134
white/mature 88
with big-size nucleus 133
with hazy cornea 133
with high myopia 89
with shallow anterior chamber 133
with small pupil 133
with weak zone 17*f*
Catching
    epinucleus sheet 179*f*
    oblique muscles 40
Cavitational effect 24
Cells
    lengthen anteriorly 4
    polishing and removal of 186*f*
Central safe zone, emulsification of piece 161*f*
Central superficial trench 98*f*
Chatter 32, 148
Chondroitin sulfate 70
Chop
    principles of 124, 124*f*
    technique 101, 121, 128
    vertical 132
Chopper 102*f*, 102, 121*f*, 145, 206*f*
    complications 135
    disadvantage of 156
    for chopping 121
    in removal of 155*f*
    misuse of 134, 156, 156*f*
    placed horizontally 136*f*
    placement of 135, 138*f*, 153
    role of 134, 153
    sharp 135*f*
    speed of 136
    types of 124, 135, 135*f*
Chopping 124, 140*f*
    completed 144*f*
    easy and safe 143*f*
    horizontal 139*f*
    of big piece 161*f*
    perfect position for horizontal 143*f*
    reverse 160*f*
    started 144*f*
    types of 124, 125*f*
        horizontal 124
        vertical 125
    without hold 133
Ciliary body 2
Classical fluid wave 77
Clear corneal
    incision 41, 52*f*, 53, 49
    main port incision 50
Coaxial irrigation-aspiration 167
    cannula 207*f*
Columnar cells, single monolayer of 4
Conjunctiva 53
    and sclera 9
Conjunctival
    chemosis 36, 40
    cutting 44
    flap 47
    incision 38
    scissors 43, 44, 202*f*
    tear 40
    thinning 9
Console 19
Continuous curvilinear capsulorhexis 71
Convex anterior capsule 71
Cornea 9, 106, 198
    hazy 62, 70, 90, 196
    mechanical injury to 163*f*
Corneal
    abrasion 40
    astigmatism 9
    epithelium 190
    haziness 12
    injury 133
    opacity 9, 46
Cortex
    blocks 176
    thin sheet of 183*f*
Cortical cataract 12
    with big-size nucleus 17*f*
Crescent 43, 44, 47, 203*f*
Crystallins
    synthesis of 4
    tend 3

Index

Cystitome 58, 60, 205*f*
    movement of 74*f*
    puncture of anterior
        capsule with 73*f*
Cytoskeleton elements 3

D

Debris 199
Deep anterior chamber 10
Deep socket 39, 191
Descemet's membrane detachment
    49, 60, 135, 173, 190, 199
Diabetes mellitus 6, 7
Dialer 102, 102*f*, 104, 113*f*, 206*f*
Dialer and chopper 104*f*, 128
    division with 105
Diamond blades 49*f*
Diaphragmatic pump 20, 21
Division
    basic instruments used for 102, 102*f*
    chopper for confirmation of 104*f*
    complications of 112
    direction of 102*f*
    ideal 105, 106*f*
    important tips related to 109
    instruments used for 103, 104*t*
    principle of 102*f*
    visco in gap of 116*f*

E

Ectoderm, surface 4
Emulsification 160*f*
    central safe zone 162*f*
    of nucleus 30
    of small pieces 30, 39, 193
Endothelial damage 32, 135
Energy 29, 80, 125, 126, 146, 147
    adequate 30
    continuous 29
    cuts 148
    modes of 148, 148*f*
        different 29, 29*f*
    role of 123, 147
    used in central zone 148
    used in empty space 148
    used in wrong way 148, 149*f*
    whitestar 30

Epinucleus 79*f*, 138*f*, 174
    and cortex, viscoexpression of 174
    edge of 180*f*
    removal of 178*f*, 182*f*
    sheet 181*f*
        remaining 183*f*
Epithelial
    cells 56*f*
    damage 135
Epithelium 2
Ethylene oxide 21
Extracapsular cataract
        extraction 37, 39, 187
    procedure 40
Eye
    hypertonic effect on 36
    movements 34
Eyeball
    normotensive 200
    control on 175
    position of 8
    primary position of 81, 101
Eyelids 9

F

Facial and retrobulbar anesthesia 35
Flared tip 24
Flat anterior capsule 57
Floppy iris syndrome 177
Flow rate, role of 147
Fluid, acoustic wave of 24
Fluidics 54
    poor 171
Foldable intraocular lens
    difficulties 190
    implantation 190, 195
    injectors for 208*f*
    relative contraindications
        for 190
Foot pedal 26, 32, 128
    correlation of hold and
        chop with 129*f*
    front view 27*f*
    functions of 123
    position 27, 28*f*, 97*f*, 123*f*, 123,
        137*f*, 137-139*f*, 142*f*, 144*f*,
        147, 168

side view 27*f*
use of 26
with parameter,
correlation of 147, 147*f*
Foot positions 124
Force, correlation of 109
Forceps
straight and curved 208*f*
used via main port 61
Foreign body, removal of 199
Funnel-shaped trench, modified 88

G

Gap holds 148
Glaucoma surgery 40
bleb of 9
Globe, horizontal position of 150
Glycolysis 3
Groove 44
superficial 110*f*
unequal 111
varies, red reflex of 84, 86*f*

H

Hastens nucleus emulsification 162*f*
Hearing, ability of 7
Heparin surface-modified lens 187
Hexose monophosphate shunt 3
Hold
principles of 122, 122*f*
variations for 132, 133*f*
Hold and chop 126
complications 133
correlation of 128
difficult situations for 134
in hemisphere 193
instruments needed for 121*f*
of nucleus 121
parameters of 125*t*, 125
procedure of 131*f*
Hold and horizontal chop,
procedure of 128
Human lens, development of 4
Hydrated lens 7
Hydro technique 195, 197

Hydrocannula beneath,
placement of 79*f*
Hydrodelamination 75, 77, 194
procedure: site of 76*f*
Hydrodelineation 75, 81, 194
procedure: site of 76*f*
sign of 78, 79*f*
Hydrodissection 75, 77, 194
cannula 206*f*
minimal or no 81
procedure: site of 76*f*
sign of 78
Hydrophilic acrylic 187
Hydrophobic acrylic 188
Hydroprocedures 75, 75*f*, 194, 196
advantages of 194
during trench 196*f*
exact location of different 194*f*
practice related to 195
Hydroxypropyl methylcellulose 69
Hypermature cataract 71
Hypermetropia 10
Hyperpulse 126, 147, 148*f*
advantages of 30
energy 30
mode 148
Hypertension 6, 7
Hypertensive retinopathy changes 7
Hyphema 192
Hypotonic, minimal 36
Hypotony 10

I

Immobile nucleus 92
Incision 41
architecture of 42, 43*f*
biplanar 50
completed by keratome 52*f*
instruments used for creation of 43
principle of 41
second side port 49
site of 46
triplanar 50
used in surgery 41
Injector system 189
Injury to anterior capsule 145

Instruments 58, 59*f*, 145
  chopper 145*f*
  phaco tip 145*f*
  used for divison
    left hand 104
    right hand 104
    types of technique 104
  viscocannula 145*f*
Intrabag manipulation 196, 197
Intraocular lens 41, 57, 191
  basic and technical aspects 187
  classification 188
    accommodative lens 188
    advance monofocal lens 188
    extended depth of focus 188
    heparin surface-modified
      lens 188
    monofocal 188
    multifocal 188
    toric lens 188
  design of 187
  foldable 188, 189
  implanting 187, 198
  in situ 198
  nonfoldable 39
  polymethyl methacrylate 187, 191
  primary 188
  secondary 188
  shape of 188
  size of 188
  types of 187
    foldable 187
    nonfoldable 187
Intuitiv machine, console of 20*f*
Iridodialysis 173
  with subsequent hyphema 177
Iris
  movement, correlation of
    incision with 54
  prolapse 173, 177, 199
    during procedure 191
  trauma 32, 135
Irrigating cannula 192
Irrigation and aspiration 33, 167, 172*f*
  cannula
    position of 175*f*
    placement of 178*f*
  design 168
  difficult 17*f*
  of epinucleus and cortex 39
  principles of 168, 169*f*
  procedure of 170, 171*f*, 172, 173*f*
  three zones for 170
  tip, direction of 170
Irrigation cannula 174*f*
Irrigation fluid, water current of 150
Ischemic heart disease 6, 7

J

Jackhammer effect 24

K

Kelman tip 8, 24, 30, 81, 85, 87*f*,
  98*f*, 158*f*
  advantage of 100*f*
  apposition of 99*f*
Keratome 38, 43, 45, 48, 52*f*, 204*f*, 208*f*
Keratometry 9
Ketamine 36
Krebs cycle 3
Kyphosis 6

L

Leathery texture cataract 7
Legion and centurion 30
Lens 11
  anatomy of 1, 5*f*
  anterior capsule of 56
  capsule 1, 2
  development of 1, 4
  epithelial cells 4
  epithelium 2
  examination of 11
  fibers 2, 3, 4
  layers of 13*f*
  loading of 190
  metabolism 3
  placode 4
  proteins 3
  single-piece 188
  three-piece 187
  with capsule, anatomy of 56*f*

Lesser instrumentation 54
Limbal
    incision 41, 44*f*
    relaxing incisions 9
    type main port incision 53
Linear 28
    mode and gradual rise 168

M

Machine, maintenance of 33
Main port and chopper 113*f*
Main port incision for 44
    limbal 44, 47
    scleral 44
McPherson forcep 207*f*
Mental intellect 7
Microcapsulorhexis forceps 58, 61, 65*f*
Microscissors 58
Microvitreoretinal 55*f*
    blade 43
Midperiphery 90
Mindset
    learning phase 91
    trench related to different 91
MVR blade 46, 48
Myopia 10

N

Nagahara chopper 135, 135*f*
    modification of 135
Neural retina 4
Nondisposable injector 189
Nuclear mass 163*f*
    catch apex of 159*f*
    hard 160*f*
Nucleus 11, 138*f*, 160*f*
    bulk of 101, 124, 126
    central hard part of 97*f*, 102*f*, 136*f*
    central part of 79*f*
    deeper layers of 79*f*
    density of 90
    depth of 111*f*
    different sizes of 14*f*
    division of 101, 193
        basic instruments used for 102
    complications 112
    different techniques 104*f*
    difficulties 112
    principle 101
    procedure 108
    special instruments used for 103
    techniques 103
    without trench 107
    drop 78*f*
    effect in central bulk of 142*f*
    energy, hard 125
    for one half of 136
    for removal of left half of 142*f*
    grading of 11, 125
    half in foot pedal position 137*f*
    halves of 130
        longitudinal axis 139*f*
    hard with small-size 15*f*
    hemispheres of 105
    left half of 132
    left side of 76
    lifting of 134
        second half of 143*f*
    management 80, 112*f*
        step in 92
    mass 158*f*, 161*f*, 165*f*
        apex of 164*f*
        catch bulk of 154*f*
        removal of 159*f*
        reorient 143*f*
        round edge of 159*f*
    piece 157
        guiding of 155
        hard part of 157
        in center 140*f*
        instruments needed for
            rotation of 128
        posterior to tip 149
        role of chopper for
            reorientation of
    posteriorly, tapping of 77*f*
    principle of 101
        division 102*f*
        rotation of 127*f*
    procedure of ideal 101
    removal of small pieces of 145, 146*f*
    right half of 130

rotation of 126, 78
rotation started 118*f*
sculpting of 80
side of 142
size of 11
trench layer-by-layer sculpting of 85*f*

O

O'Brian method 35
Opacity, site of 11
Optic nerve, damage to 36
Optic vesicle 4

P

Pain, prick 36
Palpebral fissure 8
    narrow 8, 61
Parameters 80*t*, 168
    customization of 33
    cut down 166*f*
    for removal of small pieces 147*t*
Parkinsonism 6
Peribulbar anesthesia 34, 53
Peripheral
    nucleus piece 163*f*
    piece 162*f*
Phaco
    fluidics 53, 158, 170
        understanding of 150
        with incision, correlation of 54
    handpiece 23, 23*f*
        ideal 24
    important step of 90
    in small nucleus 13*f*
    indications in 177
    machine 80
        cleaning of 28
        important terms concerned with 28
        learning 33
        parts of 19
        tubing of 22*f*
        tuning of 28
    power 29
    probe 22

    direction of 83
    entry of 38
    parts 23
    with incision, correlation of 87*f*
procedure 196
surgery 7, 19, 193, 195
    evolution of 195
    finishing steps of 191
    instruments for 201
    safe zone for 146, 146*f*
    steps of 13
time 33
    effective 33
tip 23, 23*f*, 24, 25, 102, 102*f*, 121*f*, 122, 131, 132, 139*f*, 143*f*, 145, 152, 161*f*, 163*f*, 165*f*
    and chopper 104*f*
        division with 106
        instruments 150
        used for division 117*f*
    and nucleus piece 156
    angulation of 84
    designs of 121, 122*f*
        flared aspiration of bypass system 24*f*
    direction of
        chopper toward 144*f*
        force toward 139*f*
    for emulsification of nucleus mass 162*f*
    for hold 121
    ideal placement of 153*f*
    movement of 153
    orientation of 165*f*
        nucleus pieces with
    placement of 152, 159*f*
    reoriented 142*f*
    sharpness of 80
    toward nucleus mass 162*f*
    with adequate energy 137*f*
    with different angulations 25*f*
    without chopper 162*f*
Phacoemulsification 101, 187
    machine 19
    steps in 56
    surgery
        complications 199

finishing steps in 198
procedure 198
significance 199
Polymethyl methacrylate lens, technique 191
Polypropylene 188
Port incision
first side 48
types of 53
Posterior capsule rupture 32, 145, 167, 172*f*, 190
Prechopper 104, 118*f*
deep, placement of 119*f*
horizontal placement of 120*f*
Pseudoexfoliation 10, 12, 70, 196
Pulse 147
energy 126, 148
Pump 20
peristaltic 20, 21
types of 20
Pupil
dilatation of 170
examination of 10
small 10, 90, 177, 196
Pupillary size 196

R

Rectus bridle suture, inferior 39
Rectus forcep 38
inferior 201*f*
superior 38, 201*f*
Reflux 28
Retrobulbar
anesthesia 35
hemorrhage 36
Rhexis 74*f*
size of 74*f*
speed of 74*f*
Rotation, principles of 126

S

Scleral thickness 47
Scleritis 53
Sclerocorneal incision 41
Sclerosing keratitis 53

Scoliosis 6
Senserocaine 34
Side port
ideal for division 113*f*
incision 42*f*, 45, 45*f*, 46
microvitreoretinal blade 204*f*
MVR blade angled 204*f*
Silcock needle holder 38, 201*f*
Silicone 187
lenses 187
Simcoe cannula 176, 207*f*
Sleeve 25
types of 25*f*
Slit-lamp 18*f*
cataract 13
examination 8, 11
Small capsulorhexis 133
Small nucleus, manage 13*f*
Small-incision cataract surgery 37, 39, 71, 187
conversion to 53
Sodium hyaluronate 69, 70
Soft nucleus 17*f*
Soft tissue 182*f*
aspiration of 170
bulk of 182*f*
catch bulk of 179*f*
catching apex of 178*f*
catchment 180*f*
caught 181*f*
clockwise removal of 184*f*
position of 184*f*
removal of 176
visualization 137*f*
Speculum 201*f*
Spring needle holder 208*f*
Staining, method of 62
Stitches 54
Stop and chop technique 195
Stress
minimum 197
on zonules 194
Stroke 82
length 29
Subconjunctival
anesthesia 35
hemorrhage 40

Index

Subincisional cortex
    lifting of 179*f*
    removal of 177
Subluxated cataract 89, 196
Subluxated lens 10
Sub-tenon's canula 35
Sulfated glycosaminoglycans 1
Superior rectus bridle suture 38
Surge 31
    mechanism of 31, 31*f*
Suture
    bridle 38
    tying forceps 208*f*

T

Tear
    shearing 58
    stretching 57
Teasing 160*f*
Test chamber 26, 26*f*
Tips
    aspiration port of 170
    types of 167*f*
Tissue
    apex of 168
    bulk of 168
    removal of 179*f*
    with bevel down position,
        catching of 185*f*
Tooth forcep 44, 203*f*
Torchlight examination 11
Torsional
    energy 30
    phaco
        energy 159*f*
        technology 98*f*, 158*f*
Toshniwal
    chopper 135, 135*f*
    microcapsulorhexis forcep 61, 205*f*
    prechopper 103, 103*f*, 104*f*, 107, 107*f*, 206*f*
        division by 108*f*
Transparent cells 2
Transurethral resection set 32
Trauma 8
    to iris 133

Trench 39, 80, 98*f*, 193
    adequately deep 95*f*
    center of 114*f*
    complications of 90
    depth of 86*f*
    different depth in 111*f*
    first stroke of 96*f*
    ideal 83, 101
        design of 84*f*
    illustrations of 84
    important points for 83*f*
    long 88
    on immobile nucleus 92*f*, 94*f*, 195
    related to different mindset 91*f*
    second stroke of 96*f*
    shallow 88
    start of 82*f*
    strokes of 83
    unique design of zigzag
        pattern in 85
    variation in designs of 91*f*
    visualization of base of 101
    with division, correlation of 110, 111*f*, 112*f*
Trypan blue 62
Tubing 21
    hard consistency of 22
    quality of reusable 21
Tunnel 44
Turbosonics microtip 24

U

Ultrasound energy 29
Utrata forceps 61

V

Vacuum 30, 80, 125, 126, 146, 147, 150, 168, 173
    and aspiration flow rates, role of 123
    and flow rate, minimum 185*f*
    and flow rates 81
    builds 123
    role of 147
    used in wrong way 150
Vannas scissor 58, 205*f*

Venturi pump 20
Viscocannula 102, 102*f*, 104, 104*f*, 116*f*, 117*f*, 128, 145, 156
Viscoelastic 38, 68, 145, 156, 174
    different types of 68
    removal of 191, 199
Vitreous body 1
von Lint method 35

W

Water current 152*f*
Weight instruments 113*f*
Wound
    construction of 42
        improper 177
        proper 32
    leakage 42, 192
Wrench 23, 23*f*

X

Xylocaine jelly 35

Z

Zonular dehiscence 90
Zonular dialysis 133, 168, 173, 177, 190
Zonular integrity 11
Zonular weakness 89, 196
Zonule-free area 57
Zonules 109